Medical Device Regulations Roadmap

A Beginners Guide

Des O'Brien

ISBN-13: 978-1978202955

ISBN-10: 1978202954

Contents

CHAPTER 1

INTRODUCTION

Overview of FDA structure and Key Elements

FDA's Center for Devices and Radiological Health (CDRH) is responsible for regulating firms who manufacture, repackage, relabel, and/or import medical devices sold in the United States

Medical devices are classified into Class I, II, and III. Regulatory control increases from Class I to Class III. The device classification regulation defines the regulatory requirements for a general device type. Most Class I devices are exempt from Premarket Notification 510(k); most Class II devices require Premarket Notification 510(k); and most Class III devices require Premarket Approval.

The basic regulatory requirements that manufacturers of medical devices distributed in the U.S. include the following:

- Establishment registration
- Medical Device Listing
- Premarket Notification 510(k), unless exempt, or Premarket Approval (PMA)
- Investigational Device Exemption (IDE) for clinical studies
- Quality System (QS) regulation
- Labeling requirements
- Medical Device Reporting (MDR)

Establishment Registration

Manufacturers (both domestic and foreign) and initial distributors (importers) of medical devices must register their establishments with the FDA. All establishment registrations must be submitted electronically unless a waiver has been granted by FDA. All registration information must be verified annually between October 1st and December 31st of each year. In addition to registration, foreign manufacturers must also designate a U.S. Agent. Beginning October 1, 2007

Medical Device Listing

Manufacturers must list their devices with the FDA. Establishments required to list their devices include:

- manufacturers
- contract manufacturers that commercially distribute the device
- contract sterilizers that commercially distribute the device
- repackagers and relabelers
- specification developers
- reprocessors single-use devices
- remanufacturer
- manufacturers of accessories and components sold directly to the end user
- U.S. manufacturers of "export only" devices

Premarket Notification 510(K), Unless Exempt, Or Premarket Approval (PMA)

If a device requires the submission of a Premarket Notification 510(k), the manufacturer cannot commercially distribute the device until a letter of substantial equivalence from FDA authorizing them to do so is received. A 510(k) must demonstrate that the device is substantially equivalent to one legally in commercial distribution in the United States: (1) before May 28, 1976; or (2) to a device that has been determined by FDA to be substantially equivalent.

Investigational Device Exemption (IDE) For Clinical Studies

An investigational device exemption (IDE) allows the investigational device to be used in a clinical study in order to collect safety and effectiveness data required to support a Premarket Approval (PMA) application or a Premarket Notification 510(k) submission to FDA.

Clinical studies with devices of significant risk must be approved by FDA and by an Institutional Review Board (IRB) before the study can begin.

Quality System (QS) Regulation

The quality system regulation includes requirements related to the methods used in and the facilities and controls used for: designing, purchasing, manufacturing, packaging, labeling, storing, installing and servicing of medical devices. Manufacturing facilities undergo FDA inspections to assure compliance with the QS requirements.

Manufacturers must establish and follow quality systems to help ensure that their products consistently meet applicable requirements and specifications. The quality systems for FDA-regulated products (food, drugs, biologics, and devices) are known as current good manufacturing practices (CGMP's).

The QS regulation applies to finished device manufacturers who intend to commercially distribute medical devices. A finished device is defined in 21 CFR 820.3(l) as any device or accessory to any device that is suitable for use or capable of functioning, whether or not it is packaged, labeled, or sterilized.

Certain components such as blood tubing and diagnostic x-ray components are considered by FDA to be finished devices because they are accessories to finished devices. A manufacturer of accessories is subject to the QS regulation.

FDA has determined that certain types of medical devices are exempt from GMP requirements. These devices are exempted by FDA classification regulations published in the Federal Register and codified in 21 CFR 862 to 892. Exemption from the GMP requirements does not exempt manufacturers of finished devices from keeping complaint files (21 CFR 820.198) or from general requirements concerning records (21 CFR 820.180).

Medical devices manufactured under an investigational device exemption (IDE) are not exempt from design control requirements under 21 CFR 820.30 of the QS regulation.

Labeling Requirements

Labeling includes labels on the device as well as descriptive and informational literature that accompanies the device.

Medical Device Reporting (MDR)

Incidents in which a device may have caused or contributed to a death or serious injury must to be reported to FDA under the Medical Device Reporting program. In addition, certain malfunctions must also be reported. The MDR regulation is a mechanism for FDA and manufacturers to identify and monitor significant adverse events involving medical devices. The goals of the regulation are to detect and correct problems in a timely manner.

The Medical Device Reporting (MDR) regulation (21 CFR 803) contains mandatory requirements for manufacturers, importers, and device user facilities to report certain device-related adverse events and product problems to the FDA.

Information on the requirements for each mandatory reporting group follows:

Manufacturers: Manufacturers are required to report to the FDA when they learn that any of their devices may have caused or contributed to a death or serious injury. (Key terms are defined in 21 CFR 803.3 Manufacturers must also report to the FDA when they become aware that their device has malfunctioned and would be likely to cause or contribute to a death or serious injury if the malfunction were to recur.

Importers: Importers are required to report to the FDA and the manufacturer when they learn that one of their devices may have caused or contributed to a death or serious injury. The importer must report only to the manufacturer if their imported devices have malfunctioned and would be likely to cause or contribute to a death or serious injury if the malfunction were to recur.

Device User Facilities: A "device user facility" is a hospital, ambulatory surgical facility, nursing home, outpatient diagnostic facility, or outpatient treatment facility, which is not a physician's office. User facilities must report a suspected medical device-related death to both the FDA and the manufacturer. User facilities must report a medical device-related serious injury to the manufacturer or to the FDA if the medical device manufacturer is unknown.

A user facility is not required to report a device malfunction, but can voluntarily advise the FDA of such product problems using the voluntary MedWatch Form FDA 3500 under FDA's Safety Information and Adverse Event Reporting Program.

Overview of European Regulation and Structure

An updated tranche of Regulations for medical devices and active implantable medical devices was released by the EU Commission in September 2012. The key changes as a result of new regulations include:

- Greater emphasis is placed on encouraging member state cooperation, interaction among the entities, and the use of the European database and UDI.

- European guidance (MEDDEVs) and GHTF guidance are mandatory

- Both manufacturers and Authorized Representatives must have a Qualified Person (QP)

- Expansive updates to definitions section

- Means of conformity assessment are simplified

- Notified Body requirements and functions have been revised

The definition of medical devices and active implantable medical devices covered under the MDR has being expanded to include devices that may not have a medical intended purpose, such as coloured contact lenses and cosmetic implant devices and materials. Also for inclusion within the scope of the regulation are devices designed for the purpose of "prediction" of a disease or other health condition.

Reclassification of devices according to risk, contact duration and invasiveness – The MDR will require device manufacturers to review the updated classification rules and update their technical documentation accordingly by considering the fact that class III and implantable devices will have higher clinical requirements and a regular scrutiny process.

More rigorous clinical evidence for class III and implantable medical devices – Manufacturers will need to conduct clinical investigations in case they do not have sufficient clinical evidence to support the claims done on both safety and performance of a dedicated device.

The MDR have given Notified Bodies increased post-market surveillance authority. Unannounced audits, along with product sample checks and product testing will strengthen the EU's enforcement regime and help to reduce risks from unsafe devices. Annual safety and performance reporting by device manufacturers will also be required in many cases.

This new way of regulation results in increased operating costs that draw on time and resources.

Specifications – The MDR will give the EU Commission or expert panels the authority to publish Common Specifications. These Common Specifications would exist in parallel to the Harmonised Standards and will be seen as State of the Art, and would be considered as part of the evaluation process by Notified Bodies.

Systematic clinical evaluation of Class IIa and Class IIb medical devices – Manufacturers will need to re-prepare their clinical evaluations by considering the new wording of the regulation on when an equivalence approach and under which circumstances it is possible to justify not conducting a clinical investigation.

Implementation of unique device identification – The MDR mandates the use of unique device identification (UDI) mechanisms. This requirement is expected to increase the ability of manufacturers and authorities to trace specific devices through the supply chain, and to facilitate the prompt and efficient recall of medical devices that have been found to present a safety risk. To support this effort, the European Databank on Medical Devices, (Eudamed).

Identification of "qualified person" now requires that at least one person within their organisation is ultimately responsible for all aspects of compliance with the requirements of the new MDR.

The organisation must document the specific qualifications of this individual relative to the required tasks. Further, qualifications of responsible persons will be subject to review by Notified Bodies to ensure requisite knowledge and skill.

The EU's Medical Device Regulation (MDR) came into force on 25 May 2017 and thus replacing the EU's current Medical Device Directive (93/42/EEC) and the EU's Directive on active implantable medical devices (90/385/EEC).

CHAPTER 2

DESIGN CONTROLS

Introduction

Medical devices come in all shapes and sizes with different levels of complexity and risk. They range from simple devices such as bandages, plasters and urine test strips to automated diagnostic devices, orthopaedic implants, bone screws and artificial organs. Manufacturing companies vary in size, structure, and in their approach to design, development and management practices. All of these elements influence how design controls are implemented and how effective they are. However, an understanding of the user needs, patient needs and the design control requirements is essential to all manufacturers. It leads to better project outcomes and helps foster better communication and awareness delivering a quality and product that is fit for purpose.

Design controls are a collection of practices and procedures that are incorporated into the design and development process for a product such as a medical device. It provides a structure and clear path from user needs assessment to product delivery through a step-by-step process. Design controls ensure proper assessment of the design is completed during the design and development phase. It highlights technical issues, conflicts or deficiencies in design input requirements and allows them to be addressed early on in the process. Fixing a design issue early on reduces the cost of doing so at a later point and ensures the resultant design is appropriate for its intended use. Bringing a formal review process (design control) to the table assists engineers and managers in engaging with decisions and understanding them better. It also ensures that when future changes are made, they are documented and reviewed adequately with proper consideration to the design inputs.

Design controls are a requirement of quality systems such as 21 CFR Part 820 (medical devices), and for certain classes of devices and per ISO 13485 - Quality Management Systems.

Benefits of a Design Control System:

- The intended use of the device is documented and approved
- It ensures inputs align with outputs
- It creates a design "standard" and a "process" to allow benchmarking and consistency within an organisation

Design Controls and ISO 13485 Quality Management System

Clause 7 of ISO 13485 specifies the requirements for design and development of devices as part of the product realisation process. It should be noted that organisations can opt to exclude specific requirements of ISO 13485, in cases where product realisation is not applicable. However, any such exclusion should be based on sound rationale with the technical case clearly documented. An example of this may be where design and development are not conducted by the manufacturer e.g. contract manufacturers.

Clause 7 (product realisation) of ISO 13485 details requirements for design and development controls. Clause 7 includes the following subparts:

Clause 7.1 Planning of product realisation
Clause 7.2 Customer-related processes
Clause 7.3 Design and development
Clause 7.4 Purchasing
Clause 7.5 Production and service provision
Clause 7.6 Control of measuring devices

Section 7.3 (Design and development) comprises:

Clause 7.3.1 Design and Development Planning
Clause 7.3.2 Design and Development Inputs
Clause 7.3.3 Design and Development Outputs
Clause 7.3.4 Design and Development Review
Clause 7.3.5 Design and Development Verification
Clause 7.3.6 Design and Development Validation
Clause 7.3.7 Control of Design and Development Changes

Definitions

Change Management: a management process where changes to the product, process, facilities or utilities are assessed, planned and reviewed as part of a formal systematic process.

Corrective and Preventative Action (CAPA): when an unplanned or adverse event happens, a corrective and preventative action can be implemented.

Design Phase Review: a process of evaluating the design requirements against the ability of it to deliver the intended device.

Design History File (DHF): an approved list of records that describe the design history of a medical device.

Design Input: the physical and performance requirements of a device that are the basis for the device design.

Design Output: the results of a design effort at each design phase and at the end of the total design effort. The finished design output is the basis for the device master record. The total finished design output consists of the device, its packaging and labelling, and the device master record.

Design Verification: confirmation by examination and provision of objective evidence that specified requirements have been fulfilled.

Design Validation: establishing by objective evidence that device or product specifications conform to user needs and intended use(s) defined in design documentation.

Device Master Record (DMR): a compilation of records containing the procedures and specification for a device. The contents of a DMR can contain local procedures such as SOPs and work instructions along with global or divisional specifications used to detail manufacturing processes, intermediate product or final product.

Design Phase Review: a documented, comprehensive, systematic examination of a design to evaluate the adequacy of the design requirements, the capability of the design to meet those requirements and to identify problems.

Specification: specification means any requirement to which a product, process, service, or other activity must conform.

Validation: validation means confirmation by examination and provision of objective, documented evidence that the particular requirements for a specific intended use can be consistently fulfilled.

Application of Design Controls

Design controls can be applied to any product development process. When the design input has been reviewed and the design input requirements are determined to be acceptable, the process of creating the device design begins. Product specifications are drafted and compared to the design input requirements. They then become the input for the next step in the design process. In the development and drafting of product specifications (e.g. critical quality attributes etc.) due regard must be given to product standards and industry best practices such as ISO and ASTM bodies. For example a catheter manufacturer should develop products with reference to ISO 10555 - intravascular catheters - sterile and single.

The Phase Approach to Design Control

The term "phase approach" is often used when describing the design control process. It simply means that a sequence of tasks needs to be completed, reviewed and approved during the development cycle of a product or medical device. Tasks are grouped into phases or stages. At the beginning, technical issues relating to design input requirements may need to be addressed with solutions identified. Often a range of solutions can be available, utilising different technologies. These different solutions then go on to be reviewed at the design selection process. At design selection, the project team must choose and justify a particular solution. The next phase (such as design verification and validation) ensures that the design is transferred to product launch and commercial supply - no oversights or deviations in the design intent occur. It also ensures that the device meets the user needs and intended uses (design inputs).

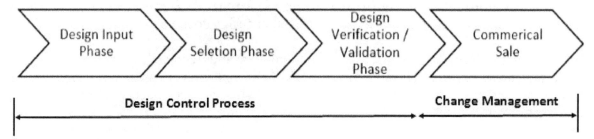

Figure: The above diagram depicts a typical product development process.

Phase Reviews Explained

A phase review is a process of evaluating the progress against the goals and activities of a particular phase. The phase review is typically completed at the end of each phase, but there may be a need to complete interim reviews for long or complex projects. For example, a design phase review is completed to ensure that the design input requirements make sense before they are interpreted into design specifications (design inputs phase review).

Managing Change

Changes made during design control are managed via document control procedures. For products built for commercial sale, the change management process is used to document and manage changes to the validated state of the process or the design of the product itself. While there may be more "flexibility" to make changes during the design phase of a project, diligence must be applied to any proposed change. Changes should be assessed by a multidisciplinary team with a management review.

Risk Management

Risk management involves the systematic application of management policies, practices and procedures that identify, analyse, control and monitor risk.

It is important to recognise that risk management should begin at the outset of the design and development phase of a project. The first step is to identify the user needs and intended use and application of the device. At the design input phase and design selection phase, risk assessments should be in a mature state. This allows the review of potential risks relating to the design of the product. Unacceptable risks can be dealt with by means of revisiting the design or introducing controls or mitigations in order to reduce the risks to acceptable levels. Following on from the design and development phase, the design verification, validation and transfer phases, or the clinical readiness phase, risk management activities and acceptability of the residual risk become the focus and must be approved indicating acceptability. This is often referred to as communicated risk.

In order to apply a risk management strategy, a procedure or SOP on risk management is typically available within manufacturing companies. This should clearly describe the risk management process and the various risk assessment tools, their application and guidance on how to complete them. The content of any risk management procedure or SOP should align with ISO 14971:2007 Medical Devices - Application of Risk Management to Medical Devices. Controlled templates for PFMEAs etc. also bring consistency and continuity to the process.

Design and Development Planning

It is the manufacturer's responsibility to establish and maintain plans that describe or reference the design and development activities and define responsibilities for implementation. The plans should identify and describe the interaction with different groups or activities that are part of the design and development process. The maintenance of plans to reflect an accurate state as the design and development progresses is also a key factor. The design and development planning is intended to be prospective in nature. It allows risks to be identified earlier and promotes timely delivery of projects.

Process Inputs and Outputs

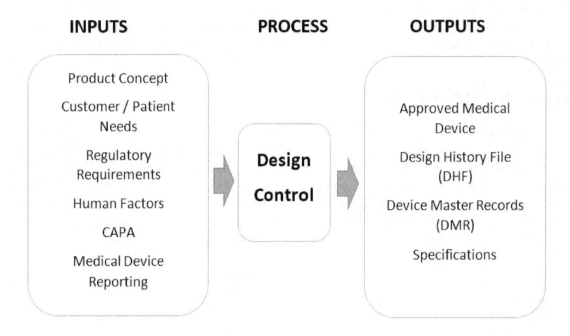

INPUTS   **PROCESS**   **OUTPUTS**

INPUTS:
Product Concept
Customer / Patient Needs
Regulatory Requirements
Human Factors
CAPA
Medical Device Reporting

PROCESS:
Design Control

OUTPUTS:
Approved Medical Device
Design History File (DHF)
Device Master Records (DMR)
Specifications

Design Input Phase

The aims of the Design Input Phase are to (1) define and document the user needs and the intended use of the medical device and (2) translate user needs and the intended use of the packaged device into design input requirements. (E.g. engineering specifications and the product requirements specifications.)

The typical documents required when establishing design inputs include:

- The creation of a formal design description detailing the intended use, user requirements and design inputs. (Note: the design description must align with the design input requirements.)
- A design and development plan which provides an estimation of timelines, resources required, responsibilities, project risks and scope of the project.
- Initial risk assessment which contains the user, design and component risks to be mitigated.
- Design concepts and technology overview.
- Business case report addressing the market size and market opportunity.

FDA 21 CFR Requirements – Design Input

21 CFR Part 820.30(C) Design Input

- Each manufacturer shall establish and maintain procedures to ensure that the design requirements relating to a device are appropriate and address the intended use of the device, including the needs of the user and patient.
- The procedures shall include a mechanism for addressing incomplete, ambiguous, or conflicting requirements.
- The design input requirements shall be documented and shall be reviewed and approved by designated individuals.

Incomplete requirements can have a serious and costly effect on the design and ultimate success of a product. If essential design requirements are omitted in error or otherwise, the impact on quality or functionality may not be detected until validation. This presents an expensive problem that may not be easily rectified. If design requirements are missed, a redesign may be necessary before a design can be released to production, thus causing delays to the project. Furthermore, if modifications are required to tooling, or process equipment, timelines can be impacted greatly. However, the safety and quality of the product must be paramount. Keeping one eye on the user requirements and intended use of the product is an important factor in avoiding gross design requirement failings.

What Is Design Input?

An artist's impression or concept documents do not meet the true intent of design input requirements. The purpose of design input is to create a complete set of requirements that are written in a technical manner with an engineering and scientific level of detail. The use of qualitative terms in a concept document is both appropriate and practical. This is often not the case for a document to be used as a basis for design. The language used in the creation of Design inputs also has a profound impact on the direction and scope of a product. If a concept document describes the product to be suitable for "outside use", then there will be requirements with regards to insulation, water ingress and operating temperatures and so on.

Scope

Design input requirements must be comprehensive. This may be quite difficult for manufacturers who are implementing a system of design controls for the first time. Design input requirements fall into three categories with most products having requirements within all three categories including:

(1) Functional requirements detailing the operation of the device.
(2) Performance requirements detailing the performance requirements or expectations of the device in relation to accuracy, speed of response times, battery life, device safety and reliability etc.
(3) Interface requirements specifying features of the device which are critical to compatibility with external systems such as the patient interface.

The scope of design input work depends on the complexity of a device and the risk associated with its use.

<u>Tips for Reviewing Design Input Requirements</u>

The ultimate goal of the design input phase is to gain agreement and approve the requirements formally. At this point, the document is a controlled document and subject to change control. Any updates required at a later date will need to be done through the change control process.

Design Input Requirements Should Be Crystal Clear: For example, a medical device may require use of a built-in battery. It would be important to specify the life expectancy of the battery. To say it has an approximate operating life of 2-3 years is too vague. A better description would be to say it has 2000 hours of operation with a software requirement that logs the number of hours the device is powered on. This mitigates the likelihood of failure during use.

Use of Tolerances: For example, a contact lens may have an outer diameter of 14.00mm. While this is the target/nominal value it cannot be ever accurately achieved. There will always be a degree of variation in the diameter measurement. Applying a tolerance, allows an acceptable range in which the measurement is within specification and accepted. If the diameter is specified as 14.00±0.2mm, designers have a basis for determining how accurate the manufacturing processes have to be. In addition, the specification will allow designers determine if the design meets the intended use.

Industry Standards: Design input requirements should meet or exceed industry standards. Compliance to product specific standards should be considered.

Regulations: Regulations that govern medical devices are mandatory. In order to supply markets, manufacturers must comply with all current regulations according to the competent authority.

Environment: The operating environment of the device should be specified. Take the example of a cardiac defibrillator. If the device is intended for use on a frontline ambulance it may be used outdoors in cold and damp conditions. On the other hand, use within a hospital setting would require greater control of the temperature range and environmental conditions.

Design Output Phase

The purpose of the design selection(output) phase is to provide a range of design options and solutions with the relevant evidence to show the effectiveness of the same. Often proof of concept (POC) or proof of principle (POP) trials may be used to verify effectiveness of solutions. POC/POP testing can involve making some limited prototypes. Any documents created in the previous phase, design input, should be reviewed and updated if required. There should be no contradictions or gaps between the documented inputs and outputs.

FDA 21 CFR Requirements – Design Output

21 CFR Part 820.30(D) Design Output

- Each manufacturer shall establish and maintain procedures for defining and documenting design output in terms that allow an adequate evaluation of conformance to design input requirements.
- Design output procedures shall contain or make reference to acceptance criteria and shall ensure that those design outputs that are essential for the proper functioning of the device are identified.
- Design output shall be documented, reviewed, and approved before release.
- The approval, including the date and signature of the individual(s) approving the output, shall be documented.

During this phase, product specifications (PS) and the device master record (DMR) are generated to define the design output. Planning for process validation and manufacturing begins during this phase often with the creation of a validation master plan (VMP). In any design office or factory setting, a lot of data and paperwork are generated. Therefore, it is important to be able to make the distinction between what is a design output and what is not. The first way of identifying a design output is to verify if it is listed as a task, a deliverable or listed in the design and development plan. If this is the case, then it is classified as a design output. Furthermore, if it describes or defines a design feature, it can also be classed as a design output.

Production Specifications

Production specifications draw upon many documents that are used to manufacture, test, inspect, install, maintain and service a device. They include: (1) component and material specifications, (2) production and process specifications, (3) work instructions and SOPs, (4) quality plans, specifications and procedures, (4) labelling specifications, and (5) packaging specifications.

Design Review

Formal design reviews are critical to the efficacy of design control, and ultimately, the market success of the device. They should be planned for up front in the design development plan. Changes late in the design cycle are much more expensive than those made early on. Design reviews can play an important role in identifying changes in a timely manner and thus prevent costly redesigns close to the launch date. The FDA QSR clearly specifies the need for independent reviewers. Independent reviewers must be far enough removed from the design in order to provide an objective review.

FDA 21 CFR Requirements- Design Review

FDA CFR Part 820.30(E) Design review

Each manufacturer shall establish and maintain procedures to ensure that formal documented reviews of the design results are planned and conducted at appropriate phases of the device's design development.

The procedures shall ensure that participants at each design review include representatives of all functions concerned with the design phase being reviewed and an individual(s) who does not have direct responsibility for the design phase being reviewed, as well as any specialists needed.

The results of a design review, including identification of the design, the date, and the individual(s) performing the review, shall be documented in the design history file (the DHF).

Key goals of design review:

- provide feedback to designers on existing or emerging problems
- assess project progress
- provide confirmation that the project is ready to move on to the next phase of development

Many types of reviews occur during the course of developing a product. Reviews may have both an internal and external focus.

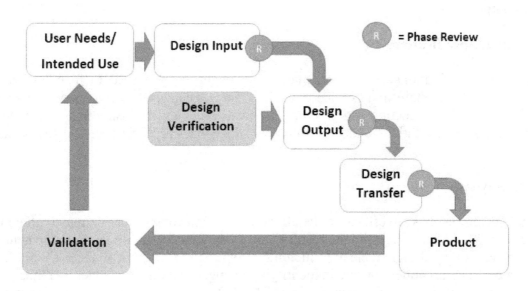

Reviews are important in ensuring that the input requirements are not forgotten as the project progresses. Secondly, there must be "agreement" between the user requirements and design inputs versus the design outputs.

Reviewers

In determining who should participate in a formal design review, planners should consider the qualifications of reviewers and the types of expertise required. Often a matrix listing reviewers, functions and responsibilities is documented in a design control procedure or at the outset of a project.

Design Verification, Validation and Transfer Phase

To illustrate the concepts, consider a building design. In a typical scenario, the senior architect establishes the design input requirements and sketches the general appearance and construction of the building, but contractors typically elaborate and interpret the details into practical terms. Verification refers to the checking at each phase to ensure the output meets the design requirements. For example, if a device is designed to take both AC electrical power and a battery (DC power), the design engineer must verify that these are accounted for in the plans and production specifications.

FDA 21 CFR Requirements - Design Verification

FDA CFR Part 820.30(f) Design Verification

- Each manufacturer shall establish and maintain procedures for verifying the device design.
- Design verification shall confirm that the design output meets the design input requirements.
- The results of the design verification, including identification of the design, method(s), the date, and the individual(s) performing the verification, shall be documented in the Design History File.

The ultimate aim of design verification is to finalise design specification. Examples of verification activities include:

- Design failure modes and effects analysis (DFMEA)
- Fault tree analysis
- Package integrity tests
- Biocompatibility testing
- Bioburden testing of packed products
- Worst case analysis – tolerance stacking of components

Design Validation

Design validation is required for the product to ensure the device meets the user requirements and intended use. Above all, it ensures the device operates reliably and safely. Process validation is required in order to confirm manufacturing specifications and the Device Master Record (DMR). However, process validation is separate to design control and is covered in Chapter 6 - Process Validation.

FDA 21 CFR Requirements - Design Validation

FDA CFR 820.30(G) Design Validation

- Each manufacturer shall establish and maintain procedures for validating the device design.
- Design validation shall be performed under defined operating conditions on initial production units, lots, batches, or their equivalents.
- Design validation shall ensure that devices conform to defined user needs, intended uses and shall include testing of production units under actual or simulated use conditions.
- Design validation shall include software validation and risk analysis, where appropriate.
- The results of the design validation, including identification of the design, method(s), the date, and the individual(s) performing the validation, shall be documented in the design history file.

Verification examines design outputs at the different phases of the process while design validation confirms that all user needs are achieved even when subject to anticipated sources of variation such as materials, processing equipment, suppliers and so on.

Design Transfer

The purpose of design transfer is to finalise all deliverables for filing with regulatory agencies.

FDA 21 CFR Requirements - Design Transfer

FDA CFR Part 820.30(H) Design Transfer

- Each manufacturer shall establish and maintain procedures to ensure that the device design is correctly translated into production specifications.

As the design output is finalised, the design is transferred into production specifications (drawings, manufacturing, test, and inspection procedures). Production specifications must ensure that manufactured devices are consistently and reliably produced within product and process capabilities, meeting all quality requirements.

Post-Launch Reviews

A post-launch review is required for each product within one year of initial launch. The purpose of the post-launch review is to confirm that no design or manufacturing changes are required and to document future product development activity. It also considers performance and patient safety.

Some post-launch activities include:

#	Action	Description
1	Post Market Surveillance	Review of data from any studies required due to conditional approval by FDA or other deliverables per Post Market Surveillance Plan
2	Product Performance Analysis	Review product complaints. Compare to equivalent devices if feasible
3	CAPA / Field	Review CAPA data. Review the severity of CAPAs and any re-occurring causes
4	Design Review	Review design or process changes since approval
5	Production Review	Yields, scrap, NCMR, causes of downtime, and any other manufacturing issues
6	Customer Feedback	review patient and user feedback

Design Control Deliverables

This section provides a non-exhaustive list of design documentation deliverables. A brief description of each is provided. This list can be used as a checklist for the design control process or as supplementary information of key activities outlined previously.

External Requirements: External requirements refer to regulations and industry standards that are relevant to a new product. At the design input phase a list of documents should be created in order to capture essential requirements as early as possible.

Design Development Plan: A design and development plan is an overarching document that describes the design and development, responsibilities, timelines and project scope, list and schedule of major tasks and the phase review details such as the timing and approval requirements.

Product Specification: The product specification is a design output document that is built over the course of the project. Not all information will be final in the early phases, however, having an early draft will help focus minds and generate the right activity in order to define target dimensions, physical attributes and tolerances.

Stability Testing: A document containing a summary of results, testing and analysis should be created and filed as part of the DHF.

Device Master Record: A DMR is an output document and should be available at the design transfer phase. It is a comprehensive list referencing all work instructions, test procedures, test specifications, manufacturing specifications and finished product specifications required to manufacture the product.

Test Method Validations: A list of all validated test methods (functional, analytical, physical etc.) should be available to file in the DHF.

Design History File: The DHF is a repository for all of the documentation generated as a result of the design control process. The DHF serves as a complete record of the design.

Design Control Process via Web-Based Systems

In recent years some companies have entered the market offering web-based design control processes. As mentioned earlier, there are a large amount of documents created during the design control process. Most of the documentation generated is subject to change control and therefore requires review and approval. As with traditional hardcopy approval, this can be time-consuming and complex if approvers are based across different departments or drawn internationally.

All documents also form part of the design history file. Therefore, the proper filing and availability of documents is an important source of concern. The use of an electronic system may mitigate some of these concerns.

Furthermore, some web-based solutions offer integration with existing electronic documentation systems or integration with quality system software such as CAPA software and/or deviation management software.

CHAPTER 3

ISO 13485

Introduction

ISO 13485 is the quality management standard of choice for manufactures of medical devices. Revised in 2016, ISO 13485:2016 "specifies requirements for a quality management system where an organisation needs to demonstrate its ability to provide medical devices and related services that consistently meet customer and applicable regulatory requirements."

The scope of the standard can apply to any organisation or company involved throughout the life-cycle of a product, including design and/or development, production, storage and distribution, installation, or servicing of a medical device and design and development or provision of technical or professional services.

The recent revision is designed to address recent developments in quality management and other updated regulations that relate to the industry. Improvements in the new version of the standard include broadening its applicability to include all organisations involved in the life cycle of the product, from the concept stage to end of life along with greater alignment with regulatory requirements and post-market surveillance including complaint handling.

ISO 13485:2016 is also used by suppliers or external vendors that provide QMS related management system- services. Requirements of ISO 13485:2016 are applicable to organisations regardless of their size and regardless of their type except where explicitly stated. Wherever requirements are specified as applying to medical devices, the requirements apply equally to associated services as supplied by the organisation. If any requirement in Clauses 6, 7 or 8 of ISO 13485:2016 is not applicable due to the activities undertaken by the organisation or the nature of the medical device for which the quality management system is applied, the organisation does not need to include such a requirement in its quality management system. For any clause that is determined to be not applicable, the organisation records the justification as part of their certification and quality management system.

The Process Approach

ISO 13485 is based on a process approach to quality management. A process is any activity that receives inputs and converts them to outputs. For an organisation to function effectively, it has to identify and manage numerous linked processes. Furthermore, many processes impact other processes or downstream processes. The application of a system of processes within an organisation, together with the identification and interactions of these processes, and their management, can be referred to as the "process approach".

Directives Versus Standards

When it comes to regulated industries such as medical devices, it is first important to be familiar with some common terms and definitions and what they really mean. This chapter examines some key terms that are applied widely and relate to regulated industries. They include:

- Directives
- Standards
- Notified Body
- Competent Authority

Directives

Directives are legal requirements which must be met by manufacturers or other bodies within the industry. Directives are based on legislation and are issued at governmental level. It is important to note that standards such as ISO 13485 help companies meet the requirements set up in directives. (See harmonised standards below)

Standards

Standards are not always mandatory. However, they help manufacturers be compliant with directives/legislation.

They also represent the current and best practice in the field of study/industry. Harmonised standards are European standards prepared under a mandate from the European Commission, referenced in the official journal, and drafted so that compliance with their requirements relates to one or more essential requirements of the directive. These standards have special status because, when a manufacturer can show that their products meet the requirements of the standard, there is a presumption that the product conforms to the essential requirements of the directive that is covered by the standard.

What is a Competent Authority?

When it comes to medical devices, a competent authority is the legally delegated authority mandated to monitor compliance to directives and legal requirements within the industry. The competent authority has the power to grant and revoke licenses.

Example of Competent Authorities:

- FDA (Food and Drug Administration) CFR Code of Federal Regulations – U.S.
- MHRA (Medicines and Healthcare Regulatory Agency - UK
- HPRA (Health Products Regulatory Agency) - Ireland
- JPAL (Japanese Regulations for Medical Devices) – Japan

What Is a Notified Body?

A notified body is a certification organisation which the national authority (the competent authority) of a member state designates to carry out one or more of the conformity assessment procedures described in the annexes of the medical devices directives. The Medicines and Healthcare Products Regulatory Agency is the UK competent authority under the three directives.

Organisations and Institutions

Many of the common acronyms that are referenced in literature relate to various standard setting organisations and industry representatives. Some of the more common bodies are listed below:

ISO: Internal Organisation for Standardisation
IMDR (F): International Medical Device Regulators Forum
ASTM: American Society for Testing and Materials
GHTF: Global Harmonisation Task Force

Basic Definitions (Source: Annex IX of Directive 93/42/EEC)

Intended Purpose: Intended purpose means the use for which the device is intended according to the data supplied by the manufacturer on the labelling, in the instructions and/or in promotional materials. (Chapter I section 1 of Annex IX of Directive 93/42/EEC)

Transient: Normally intended for continuous use for less than 60 minutes.

Short Term: Normally intended for continuous use for not more than 30 days.

Long Term: Normally intended for continuous use for more than 30 days.

Invasive Devices: A device which, in whole or in part, penetrates inside the body, either through a body orifice or through the surface of the body.

Body Orifice: Any natural opening in the body, as well as the external surface of the eyeball, or any permanent artificial opening, such as a stoma.

Surgically Invasive Device: An invasive device which penetrates inside the body through the surface of the body, with the aid of or in the context of a surgical operation.

Implantable Device: Any device which is intended:

- to be totally introduced into the human body or,

- to replace an epithelial surface or the surface of the eye, by surgical intervention which is intended to remain in place after the procedure. Any device intended to be partially introduced into the human body through surgical intervention and intended to remain in place after the procedure for at least 30 days is also considered an implantable device.

Medical Device: means any instrument, apparatus, appliance, material or other article, whether used alone or in combination, together with any accessories or software for its proper functioning, intended by the manufacturer to be used for human beings in the:

- diagnosis, prevention, monitoring, treatment or alleviation of disease or injury.
- investigation, replacement or modification of the anatomy or of a physiological process.
- control of conception which does not achieve its principal intended action by pharmacological, chemical, immunological or metabolic means.

A medical device may be assisted in its function by the following means:

Active Medical Device: any medical device relying for its functioning on a source of electrical energy or any source of power other than that directly generated by the human body or gravity.

Active Implantable Medical Device: any active medical device which is intended to be totally or partially introduced, surgically or medically, into the human body or by medical intervention into a natural orifice, and which is intended to remain after the procedure.
Custom-Made Device: means any active implantable medical device specifically made in accordance with a medical specialist's written prescription which gives, under his responsibility, specific design characteristics and is intended to be used only for an individual named patient.

Device Intended for Clinical Investigation: any active implantable medical device intended for use by a specialist doctor when conducting investigations in an adequate human clinical environment.
Intended Purpose: means the use for which the medical device is intended and for which it is suited according to the data supplied by the manufacturer in the instructions.

Putting into Service: means making available to the medical profession for implantation.

Where an active implantable medical device is intended to administer a substance defined as a medicinal product within the meaning of Council Directive 65/65/EEC of 26 January 1965 on the approximation of provisions laid down by law, regulation or administrative action relating to proprietary medicinal products (6), as last amended by Directive 87/21/EEC (7), that substance shall be subject to the system of marketing authorisation provided for in that directive.

Where an active implantable medical device incorporates, as an integral part, a substance which, if used separately, may be considered to be a medicinal product within the meaning of Article 1 of Directive 65/65/EEC, that device must be evaluated and authorised in accordance with the provisions of this directive.

ISO 13485 & Regulations

In Europe, EN ISO 13485:2013 helps companies meet the requirements of: Directive 93/42/EEC on medical devices. This harmonised standard gives companies the "presumption of conformity" to complying with directives.

EN ISO 13485 was published in February 2013 and harmonised in August 2013 to cover the three directives:

- 90/385/ECC– The Active Implantable Medical Devices Directive (AIMDI)
- 93/42/ECC – The Medical Devices Directive (MDD)
- 98/79/EEC – In Vitro Diagnostic MDD (IVDMDD)

In the United States, medical device manufacturers need to meet the requirements of 21 CFR Part 820 of FDA regulations. While ISO 13485 is not an actual requirement, many companies will seek certification to the standard to support the exporting of products.

In Australia, it is a regulatory requirement for manufacturers of medical devices to meet the requirements of ISO 13485. In Canada, certification to ISO13485 is part of the regulatory requirements. The content of ISO 13485 is interpretive (not prescriptive) which gives a degree of scope in how the requirements are applied and met within a company. ISO 13485 provides both a sound and widely recognised basis in meeting regulatory compliance for medical devices. Based off ISO 19001 however, ISO 13485 is a standalone standard for medical devices.

ISO 9001 has requirements and themes relating to continual improvement and customer satisfaction. These have been modified for ISO 13485.

Main differences between ISO 9001 & ISO 13485:

• Customer satisfaction is changed to customer feedback
• Extra requirements regarding procedures for ISO 13485
• Extra requirements for records ISO 13485 (e.g. retention)
• Continual improvement is restricted to continual improvement of the quality management system

ISO 13485 has extra requirements required for regulatory bodies such as post production review and management of advisory events.

ISO 13485 and ISO/TR 14969

ISO/TR 14969 is a technical report that is used for guidance on the application and implantation of ISO 13485. It is recommended for those responsible for the role out of ISO 13485 within their organisation. The content of ISO/TR 14969 is based on several established organisations such as the GHTF, ISO and input from regulatory bodies.

Standard Overview

ISO 13485 has 8 Clauses or Sections which make up the structure of the standard.

Section 0 Normative References, Definitions and Terms
Section 1 Requirements of the Quality Management System (QMS)
Section 2 Normative References
Section 3 Terms and Definitions
Section 4 Requirements of the Quality Management System (QMS)
Section 5 Management Responsibility
Section 6 Resource Management
Section 7 Product Realisation
Section 8 Measurement, Analysis and Improvement

CLAUSE 1: SCOPE

This section refers to the scope and application of the standard.

- The organisation must be able to show its ability to provide medical devices to meet customer requirements and regulatory requirements
- A key aim of the standard is to allow harmonisation to regulatory requirements
- The scope of the QMS must relate to medical devices for a company to be able to use ISO 13485

Some examples of what's in scope of the standard include (1) the manufacture of hip implants, (2) the design and manufacturing of in-vitro blood testing devices, (3) contact analytical testing (4) consultancy services. The terms "where appropriate" and "if appropriate" are used throughout the standard, therefore, it should be met by the organisation unless a justification is documented.

CLAUSE 2: NORMATIVE REFERENCES

This clause states that when working with ISO 13485; refer to ISO 9000:2000 for fundamentals and vocabulary.

CLAUSE 3: TERMS AND DEFINITIONS

This clause provides terms and definitions. It is very useful in the early days of establishing and implementing ISO 13485 to ensure that terms and definitions are clearly understood.

CLAUSE 4: QUALITY MANAGEMENT SYSTEM

Clause 4 details the general requirements that relate to the quality management system, the documentation requirements and record requirements.

Clause 4 includes:
4.1 General requirements clause
4.2 Documentation requirements clause

CLAUSE 4.1 GENERA REQUIREMENTS

The organisation must implement a Quality Management System, or QMS in order to provide the framework and structure to achieve ISO 13485 roll-out and implementation. However, the role of the QMS does not stop there. After initial roll-out, the requirements of the standard must be maintained and determined to be effective on an on-going basis. The following processes should be documented:

- List of all processes
- Process interactions
- Monitoring of processes
- Resources to facilitate rollout of processes
- Measure and monitor effectiveness
- System of identifying improvements

CLAUSE 4.2: DOCUMENTATION REQUIREMENTS

When it comes to the regulated industries such as the medical device industry, every process and procedure must be documented. Documentation ensures that everyone is working in the same manner with the same procedures. However, documentation is more than just writing down procedures and processes. It is also concerned with how documents are controlled, how they are updated and how they are stored.

Electronic Document Management Systems

Electronic document management systems aka EDMS are now the norm and gold standard for most medium to large organisations. Many companies that provide medical device manufacturers with an EDMS can customise the system to match the business processes particular to an organisation. With configurable or customisable software, validation and proper verification is important to ensure the system operates as intended. There are also regulatory requirements that stipulate the expectations and requirements of such systems. For example, the application of electronic signatures and the presence of audit trials. FDA 21 CRF Part 11 details the requirements with regards to electronic records and electronic signatures. For medicinal products in Europe, GMP V4 Annex 11 specifies similar requirements.

Changes and Updates to Documents

Revision control is a key element of the Quality Management Systems in place in regulated industries. As the need for changes in the document arises, the controlled document can be amended/updated. With each update the version number revises also. Some companies will use alphabetic revision control and to a lesser extent numeric revision control (Version A, Version B or Version 01, Version 02).
Controlled documents should always have a version number or revision number electronically on each page of the document. This is similar to books which always list what edition they are. E.g. first edition or second edition.

Records

Records are generated through the application of processes and procedures. These records can be related in quality inspection and manufacturing. The integrity and quality of records relating to the manufacture of medical devices is important, as it plays a part in safe-guarding the patient or user. Records may also help in the investigation of any quality issues, complaints or adverse events that may arise.

Principles of Good Documentation Practices or GDP, should be applied to records. In particular, handwritten entries should always be accompanied by a signature and date. This is important as traceability must be maintained in the event of an issue or complaint.

CLAUSE 5: MANAGEMENT RESPONSIBILITY

Clause 5 includes:

5.1 Management Commitment
5.2 Customer Focus
5.3 Quality Policy
5.4 Planning
5.5 Responsibility, Authority and Communication
5.6 Management Review

5.1 Management Commitment

It is essential that top management have an authentic and tangible commitment to meeting regulations and the expectations of customers. Quality should be at the forefront of all of activities. Management should encourage discourse and communication on all matters relating to internal processes, quality and the QMS as a whole.

5.2 Customer Focus

Customer feedback is a requirement of ISO 13485 and as such the manufacturer must engage with the customer. In instances where a defective product is received, the manufacturer must have a complaints process to facilitate proper feedback, communication and investigation.

5.3 Quality Policy

Simple statement /1 pager or more
Often quality policies will be displayed in reception areas etc. Copies should be signed and revision controlled.

Quality policy must have a commitment to maintain the effectiveness of the QMS.

5.4 Planning

Top management must plan quality objectives and ensure they are implemented and effective. Some examples of quality objectives include:

- reduce rework by 10%
- reduce scrap by 5%
- have customer complaints reduced by 2% per year

5.5 Responsibility, Authority and Communication

- Roles and responsibilities are defined
- Job descriptions are in place
- Organisational charts are in place and accurate

5.6 Management Review

The purpose of management review is to ensure the effectiveness of the QMS.
Inputs to management review include:

(a) Audit results

(b) Customer feedback
(c) Process performance and conformity
(d) Corrective and preventative actions
(e) Deviations
(f) Regulatory changes and revisions

CLAUSE 6: RESOURCE MANAGEMENT

Clause 6 of ISO 13485 is concerned with human resources, infrastructure and work environment.
Clause 6 includes:

6.2 Human resources
6.3 Infrastructure
6.4 Work Environment

People are the key part of any QMS. Therefore, they should have the appropriate level of education, skill and experience. A culture of quality must be lived by everyone.

People must be suitably trained. Training must be documented and consistent throughout an organisation. Training must be seen to be effective. Proper records of education and training must be kept.

Human intelligence, human creativity and human labour are all key inputs to any factory or company manufacturing medical devices. Therefore, an organisation must be properly resourced in order to function correctly, meet the regulatory requirements and customer expectations.

6.2 Human resources

"Change the people or change the people"

With any organisation, it is only as good as the people it has in its make-up. Therefore, the people, operators, engineers, managers etc. all contribute to the quality management system. Clause 6.2.2 also specifies requirements with regards to competence, awareness and training. The person should be matched to the job in terms of their qualifications, experience and training. Typically, job descriptions are used to drive and capture these requirements. Nowadays, most multinational companies will ask for evidence of qualifications, training and experience. These documents are then held on file in the event of an audit. This is recommended practice for medical device companies. While the standard does not specifically call out the need to hold records of degrees and qualifications on file, the company or organisation needs to demonstrate the suitability of the person to their respective roles, and filing the qualification provides the easiest method.

6.3 Infrastructure

Infrastructure has the ability to impact the quality of products and services. Therefore, it must be fit for purpose. It is especially important if the organisation is involved with the manufacture of medical devices. The following element need to be considered with regards to infrastructure:

- Location of equipment and the operating environment
- Equipment installation and validation
- Utilities required for the operation of equipment and systems
- Layout of the factory – flow or raw materials, in-process materials and finished products
- Environmental systems such as HVAC and fire suppression systems

6.4 Work Environment

The work environment is also closely related to infrastructure within a given organisation and they can both affect or impact upon the quality of products manufactured. Risk to product quality and patients is minimised by understanding the work environment and how it can impact the product. When the interactions and risks are understood, work can then be done to eliminate risks or at least control or monitor them. Environmental conditions that can impact upon product quality include:

- Humidity
- Temperature
- Air quality
- Room pressure differentials (negative / positive)
- Air flow/velocity

CLAUSE 7: PRODUCT REALISATION

Clause 7 includes:

7.1 Planning of product realisation
7.2 Customer-related processes
7.3 Design and development
7.4 Purchasing
7.5 Production and service provision
7.6 Control of measuring devices
7.1 Planning of Product Realisation

Product realisation can be defined as a collection of processes and body of work that delivers a product or service to the customer. Remember, when it comes to medical devices, customers can be patients or users such as doctors and nurses. It should be noted that organisations can opt to exclude specific requirements, in cases where product realisation is not applicable. However, any such exclusion should be based on sound rationale with the case clearly documented. An example of this may be where design and development is not conducted by the manufacturer e.g. contract manufacturers.

7.1 Planning of Product Realisation

Planning is an often underestimated but remains a key element of product realisation. If adequate time and resources are given to planning, it makes all other processes run smoother, and therefore should help to produce improved products and services.

7.2 Customer-Related Processes

There are 3 elements that feed into customer-related processes. They include the following:
Determining the requirements related to the product Clause 7.2.1
Review of requirements relating to the product-Clause 7.2.2
Customer communication-clause 7.2.3

Customer requirements are typically captured in a User Requirements Specification. A requirements specification (URS) documents all of the desired attributes of a product or service. They can be made up by a combination of CQAs, regulatory requirements and design requirements. A URS can then form the basis for review of the product or service requirements.
With regard to customer communication, it is important to remind ourselves that we are concerned with ISO 13485 which as we very well know by now is the standard for medical devices. Therefore, having the right information available to the customer, patient or end user is important. When additional information needs to be transmitted or updates to information need to be communicated, an advisory note can be issued. Another important aspect of customer communication is customer feedback. This communication can be made up of positive feedback from the customer or users, or when there is a query with regard to a product or service. Therefore, processes or systems must be in place to make communication between customer and company both effective and timely.

7.3 Design and Development

Design and Development Verification and Validation ensure that the product is designed, developed and subsequently manufactured meeting all the customer requirements, regulatory requirements and business requirements. These requirements are classed as inputs to the design and development, and verification and validation ensure the inputs have been adequately taken into account.

The design and development testing sometimes replicate the commercial applications of the medical device, hence providing a realistic challenge in order to have confidence in the medical device.

Design Control

Design control is a necessary practice that ensures good engineering principles are maintained throughout the design phase of a product. It also refers to the continual design and development of the product through its very lifecycle. The design and development files and history must be controlled and maintained, with any changes properly assessed, tested and documented.

7.4 Purchasing

Bearing in mind that a quality management system considers all aspects of an organisation's functioning, purchasing and procurement of materials necessitates putting robust controls in place. Simply put, a purchasing process must exist.

7.5 Production and Service Provision

This requirement of ISO 13485 is an extensive section with a great deal of importance associated with it. As we are dealing with the manufacture of medical devices (or other activity associated with medical devices) there are specific requirements for sterile products. If a product is sterile, its use or application is likely to be associated with greater risks to the patient. Therefore, extra safeguards must be in place for sterile medical devices. Key sections of Clause 7.5 include: (1) control of production and service provision – both general and specific requirements, (2) specific requirements for sterile medical devices, (3) validation of equipment and processes for production and service provision, (4) traceability and identification, (5) preservation of product controls with regard to monitoring and measuring medical devices.

7.6 Control of Measuring Devices

This clause requires an organisation to identify what monitoring and measuring is required and to ensure the product or service meets the customer requirements. A calibration procedure must also be maintained to ensure the equipment is accurate and reliable. Calibration must ensure that:

- Equipment used to verify product quality is calibrated to a periodic schedule.
- The calibration is performed to an international standard.
- The calibration status of the equipment is recorded and visible.
- The equipment must be located within a suitable area in order to maintain accurate and reliable results.

If an organisation uses any computer software to monitor or measure outputs, the software must be verified before use via the appropriate validation and qualification activities.

CLAUSE 8: MEASUREMENT ANALYSIS

Clause 8 includes:
8.1 General requirements
8.2 Monitoring and measurement
8.3 Control of nonconforming products
8.4 Analysis of data
8.5 Improvement

8.1 General Requirements

Measurement, analysis and improvement are the key themes of clause 8. As with all medical devices, inspection and testing both during manufacturing and post manufacturing is necessary to ensure products and services function as intended and without defects. With any type of measurement or inspection analysis, the method used to complete the testing is critical. The method must be fit for purpose, and the equipment must be suitable. This "method validation" typically is done during the design and development phase.

8.2 Monitoring and Measurement

Monitoring and measurement are dependent on the information or feedback provided from various sources. The most important feedback is the post-production feedback that is gathered from customers or the end user. Again, this occurs over the whole lifetime of the product or service in question. There are a number of methods that can be used to obtain feedback. Some examples include:

-Customer surveys
-Customer complaints
-Review of regulatory databases such as MAUDE.
-Repair and servicing information

8.3 Control of Nonconforming Product

Non-conforming product presents a risk to patients or users of medical devices. When a situation arises where non-conforming product is manufactured or detected through inspection processes, the product must be controlled and segregated to prevent unintended use or distribution.
Some examples resulting in non-conformance are:

- When a manufacturing process drifts outside its validation window or operating parameters.

- A certificate of analysis for a raw material is not provided by the supplier or the results are out of specification.
- In-process testing was not completed at the defined intervals.
- Training of personnel completing tests is not current or is inadequate.

8.4 Analysis of Data

In any engineering activity, data and the quality of the data is a key factor in making the right decisions. Provided the data collected is relevant and accurate, analysis of data can provide important insights into process performance, quality control and product functionality. Data should be collated in a consistent way and controlled by a procedure. When it comes to medical device manufacturing, the sources and types of data are multiple. Data can be generated from in-process testing and data can be generated from end of line testing aka finished product testing.

8.5 Improvement

ISO 13485 fosters a culture of continual improvement. As we have seen, each activity can be described as a process. For example, a manufacturing process, a procurement process, a complaints process. The set of processes that make up the quality management system need to be continually reviewed to ensure they are suitable and effective for the task at hand. Typical tools used to keep improvement in mind include:

- Review of the quality policy and quality objectives
- Frequency and category of corrective and preventative actions (CAPA's)
- Customer complaints
- Management review input

CE Marking

In Europe a QMS is required for CE marking of a medical device that is placed on the market in the EU.

ISO 13485:2003 is a harmonised standard that can be used by companies to show conformity of their QMS to requirements of directives. EN ISO 13485:2012 was harmonised in August 2012. This allows compliant companies receive an EC Declaration of Conformity.

Summary of the CE Requirements

Manufacturers of class I devices or their authorised representatives must:

- review the classification rules to confirm that their products fall within class I (Annex IX of the Directive)
- check that their products meet the essential requirements (Annex I of the Directive)

- notify the competent authority, in advance, of any proposals to carry out a clinical investigation to demonstrate safety and performance of a device as required by the regulations
- obtain notified body approval for sterility or metrology aspects of their devices and where applicable prepare relevant technical documentation
- Draw up the 'EC Declaration of Conformity' (below) before applying the CE marking to their devices
- Register with the competent authority
- Implement and maintain corrective action and vigilance procedures including a systematic procedure to review experience gained in the post-production phase
- Make available relevant documentation on request for inspection by the competent authority.

In Europe, all medical devices must bear the CE marking of conformity (see Annex XII) of the directive) when they are placed on the market and/or put into service. The CE marking must appear in a visible, legible and indelible form on the device or its sterile pack, where practicable and appropriate, and where applicable on any instructions for use and sales packaging. For 'sterile' and 'measuring' devices, the CE marking must be accompanied by the identification number of the notified body that has acted under the relevant conformity assessment procedure.

EC Declaration of Conformity

In order to affix the CE marking, the manufacturer or their authorised representative must follow the EC declaration of conformity procedure referred to in Annex VII of the directive. This procedure must be completed prior to placing the device on the market. The 'EC declaration of conformity' is the procedure whereby the manufacturer or their authorised representative prepares the required technical documentation, puts into place corrective action and vigilance procedures and declares that the products meet the requirements set out in the directive.

Technical Documentation

The technical documentation should be prepared following review of the essential requirements and must cover all of the following aspects:

Description: A general description of the product, including any variants (for example names, model numbers and sizes).

Raw Materials and Component Documentation: Specifications including, as applicable, details of raw materials, drawings of components and/or master patterns and any quality control procedures.
Intermediate Product and Sub-Assembly Documentation: Specifications including appropriate drawings and/or master patterns, circuits, and formulation specification; relevant manufacturing methods and any quality control procedures.

Packaging and Labelling Documentation: Packaging specifications and copies of all labels and any instructions for use.

Design Verification: The results of qualification tests and design calculations relevant to the intended use of the product, including connections to other devices in order for it to operate as intended.

Risk Analysis: The results of risk analysis to review whether any risks associated with the use of the product are compatible with a high level of protection of health and safety and are acceptable when weighed against the benefits to the patient or user. If biocompatibility is relevant – for example for skin contact and invasive devices – a compilation and review of existing data or test reports based on the relevant standards is required.

Compliance with the Essential Requirements and Harmonised Standards: A list of relevant harmonised standards (for example sterilisation, labelling and information, biocompatibility, electrical safety, risk analysis, product group standards) which have been applied in full or in part of the products. If relevant harmonised standards have not been applied in full, then additional data will be required, detailing the solutions adopted to meet the relevant essential requirements of the directive. The manufacturer may choose to prove conformity with the essential requirements of the directive through the use of their own standards and/or other relevant published standards (ISO, EN, BS). However, the use of such standards does not give similar, immediate presumption of conformity to the essential requirements of the directive. Therefore, using a harmonised standard provides greater protection to the manufacturer.

Device Classification

The manufacturer, in preparing for CE marking, should first determine if their product falls within the scope of the directive or national regulation, either as a medical device or as an accessory to a medical device, as defined in Article 1 of directive 93/42/EEC and Article 2 of the regulation. In order to be classified as a medical device, the product should have a medical purpose and its primary mode of action will typically be physical.

Level of Risk

General medical devices and related accessories must be classified into one of four classes, which are based on the perceived risk of the device to the patient or user. The classification of a device determines the conformity assessment options that are applicable to the device, with higher risk devices undergoing higher levels of assessment.

Class   Risk level

I	Low Risk
IIa	Medium Risk
IIb	Higher Risk
III	Highest Risk

Classification Rules

There are eighteen rules outlined in Annex IX of the directive and related regulation that lay down the basic principles of classification. In MEDDEV 2.4/1 Rev. 8, these rules are further explained and descriptive examples are provided. The eighteen rules are subdivided into four groups as follows:

Rules	**Device Type**
Rules 1 – 4	Non-invasive Devices
Rules 5 – 8	Invasive Devices
Rules 9 – 12	Active Devices
Rules 13-18	Special Rule e.g. devices containing tissue of animal origin, drug-device combinations

Annex IX and related guidance documents outline a number of key characteristics, listed below, that must be considered to correctly classify a device using the eighteen classification rules:

General Principles of Device Classification

o Medical devices are defined as articles which are intended to be used for a medical purpose. It is the intended purpose that determines the class of device and not the particular technical characteristics of the device. The intended purpose of the device should be substantiated (if required) and be representative of the technical characteristics of the device.
o It is the intended and not the accidental use of the device that determines its class.
o It is the intended purpose assigned by the manufacturer to the device that determines the class of device and not the class assigned to other similar products.
o Accessories are classified separately from their parent device.
o The mode of action of a medical device should be clear and evidenced with appropriate data to confirm this mode of action.
o If the device can be classified according to several rules then the highest possible class applies.
o Multipurpose equipment which may be used in combination with medical devices are not themselves classed as medical devices unless the manufacturer places them on the market with the specific intended purpose as a medical device.
o If the device is not intended to be used solely or principally in a specific part of the body, it must be considered and classified on the basis of the most critical specified use.

Summary Of Rules

(Source: Guidelines Relating To The Application Of
The Council Directive 93/42/EEC On Medical Devices, MEDDEC 2.4/Rev.9 June 2010)

Rule 1

Rule 1: All non-invasive devices are in Class I, unless one of the other 17 rules apply. This is a fallback rule applying to all devices that are not covered by a more specific rule.
This is a rule that applies in general to devices that come into contact only with intact skin or that do not touch the patient.
Some non-invasive devices are indirectly in contact with the body and can influence internal physiological processes by storing, channeling or treating blood, other body liquids or liquids which are returned or infused into the body or by generating energy that is delivered to the body. These must be excluded from the application of this rule and be handled by another rule because of the hazards inherent in such indirect influence on the body.

Rule 2

Rule 2: All non-invasive devices are in Class I, unless one of the other 17 rules apply.

These types of devices must be considered separately from the non-contact devices of Rule 1 because they may be indirectly invasive. They channel or store substances that will eventually be administered to the body. Typically these devices are used in transfusion, infusion, extracorporeal circulation and delivery of anaesthetic gases and oxygen.

In some cases devices covered under this rule are very simple gravity activated delivery devices.

Rule 2: All non-invasive devices intended for channelling or storing blood, body liquids or tissues, liquids or gases for the purpose of eventual infusion, administration or introduction into the body are in Class IIa:

- if they may be connected to an active medical device in Class IIa or a higher class,

-if they are intended for use for storing or channelling blood or other body liquids or for storing organs, parts of organs or body tissues.

- in all other cases they are in Class I.

Rule 3

Rule 3: Non-invasive devices that modify biological or chemical composition of blood, body liquids or other liquids intended for infusion into the body.

These types of devices must be considered separately from the non-contact devices of Rule 1 because they are indirectly invasive. They modify substances that will eventually be infused into the body. This rule covers mostly the more sophisticated elements of extracorporeal circulation sets, dialysis systems and autotransfusion systems as well as devices for extracorporeal treatment of body fluids which may or may not be immediately reintroduced into the body, including, where the patient is not in a closed loop with the device.

Rule 3: All non-invasive devices intended for modifying the biological or chemical composition of blood, other body liquids or other liquids intended for infusion into the body are in Class IIb,
unless the treatment consists of filtration, centrifugation or exchange of gas or heat, in which case they are in Class IIa.

These devices (Rule 3) are normally used in conjunction with an active medical device covered under Rule 9 or Rule 11.

Filtration and centrifugation should be understood in the context of this rule as exclusively mechanical methods.

Rule 4

Rule 4: Non-invasive devices which come into contact with injured skin. This rule is intended to primarily cover wound dressings independently of the depth of the wound. The traditional types of products, such as those used as a mechanical barrier, are well understood and do not result in any great hazard. There have also been rapid technological developments in this area, with the emergence of new types of wound dressings for which non-traditional claims are made, e.g. management of the micro-environment of a wound to enhance its natural healing mechanism.

More ambitious claims relate to the mechanism of healing by secondary intent, such as influencing the underlying mechanisms of granulation or epithelial formation or preventing contraction of the wound. Some devices used on breached dermis may even have a life-sustaining or lifesaving purpose, e.g. when there is full thickness destruction of the skin over a large area and/or systemic effect. Dressings containing medicinal products which act ancillary to the dressing fall within Class III under Rule 13.

Rule 4: All non-invasive devices which come into contact with injured skin:

- are in Class I if they are intended to be used as a mechanical barrier, for compression or for absorption of exudates,
- are in Class IIb if they are intended to be used principally with wounds which have breached the dermis and can only heal by secondary intent.

Products covered under this rule are extremely claim sensitive, e.g. a polymeric film dressing would be in Class IIa if the intended use is to manage the micro-environment of the wound or in Class I if its intended use is limited to retaining an invasive cannula at the wound site. Consequently it is impossible to say a priori that a particular type of dressing is in a given class without knowing its intended use as defined by the manufacturer. However, a claim that the device is interactive or active with respect to the wound healing process usually implies that the device is in Class IIb.

Most dressings that are intended for a use that is in Class IIa or IIb, also perform functions that are in Class I, e.g. that of a mechanical barrier. Such devices are nevertheless classed according to the intended use in the higher class.

For such devices incorporating a medicinal product or a human blood derivative see Rule 13 or animal tissues or derivatives rendered non-viable see Rule 17.

Rule 5

Rule 5: Devices invasive with respect to body orifices.

Invasiveness with respect to the body orifices (ear, mouth, nose, eye, anus, urethra and vagina) must be considered separately from invasiveness that penetrates through a cut in the body surfaces (surgical invasiveness). For short term use, a further distinction must be made between invasiveness with respect to the less vulnerable anterior parts of the ear, mouth and nose and the other anatomical sites that can be accessed through natural body orifices.

Surgically created stoma, which for example allows the evacuation of urine or faeces, should also be considered as a body orifice.

Devices covered by this rule tend to be diagnostic and therapeutic instruments used in particular specialities (ENT, ophthalmology, dentistry, proctology, urology and gynaecology).

Rule 5: All invasive devices with respect to body orifices, other than surgically invasive devices and which are not intended for connection to an active medical device or which are intended for connection to an active medical device in Class I:

- are in Class I if they are intended for transient use,
- are in Class IIa if they are intended for short term use
except if they are used in the oral cavity as far as the pharynx, in an ear canal up to the ear drum or in a nasal cavity , in which case they are in Class I,
- are in Class IIb if they are intended for long term use,
except if they are used in the oral cavity as far as the pharynx, in an ear canal up to the ear drum or in a nasal cavity and are not liable to be absorbed by the mucous membrane, in which case they are in Class IIa.

All invasive devices with respect to body orifices, other than surgically invasive devices, intended for connection to an active medical device in Class IIa or a higher class, are in Class IIa.

Rule 6

Rule 6: Surgically invasive devices intended for transient use (< 60 minutes)
This rule primarily covers three major groups of devices: devices that are used to create a conduit through the skin (needles, cannulae, etc.), surgical instruments (scalpels, saws, etc.) and various types of catheters, suckers, etc.

This rule primarily covers three major groups of devices: devices that are used to create a conduit through the skin (needles, cannulae, etc.), surgical instruments (scalpels, saws, etc.) and various types of catheters, suckers, etc.

Rule 6: All surgically invasive devices intended for transient use are in Class IIa unless they are:
-intended specifically to control, diagnose, monitor or correct a defect of the heart or of the central circulatory system through direct contact with these parts of the body, in which case they are in Class III
-reusable surgical instruments, in which case they are in Class I

-intended specifically for use in direct contact with the central nervous system, in which case they are in Class III,

- intended to supply energy in the form of ionising radiation in which case they are in Class IIb,

- intended to have a biological effect or to be wholly or mainly absorbed in which case they are in Class IIb,

- intended to administer medicines by means of a delivery system, if this is done in a manner that is potentially hazardous taking account of the mode of application, in which case they are Class IIb.

Rule 7

Rule 7: Surgically invasive devices intended for short-term use (>60 minutes, <30 days). These are mostly devices used in the context of surgery or post-operative care (e.g. clamps, drains), infusion devices (cannulae, needles) and catheters of various types.

Rule 7: All surgically invasive devices intended for short term use are in Class IIa unless they are intended:

- either specifically to control, diagnose, monitor or correct a defect of the heart or of the central circulatory system through direct contact with these parts of the body, in which case they are in Class III,

- or specifically for use in direct contact with the central nervous system, in which case they are in Class III,

- or to supply energy in the form of ionising radiation in which case they are in Class IIb,
- intended to have a biological effect or to be wholly or mainly absorbed in which case they are in Class III, - or to undergo chemical change in the body, except if the devices are placed in the teeth, or to administer medicines, in which case they are Class IIb.

Rule 8

Rule 8: Implantable devices and long-term surgically invasive devices (> 30 days). These are mostly implants in the orthopaedic, dental, ophthalmic and cardiovascular fields as well as soft tissue implants such as implants used in plastic surgery.

Rule 8: All implantable devices and long-term surgically invasive devices are in Class IIb unless they are intended:
- to be placed in the teeth, in which case they are in Class IIa,
- to be used in direct contact with the heart, the central circulatory system or the central nervous system, in which case they are Class III,
- to have a biological effect or to be wholly or mainly absorbed, in which case they are in Class III,
- or to undergo chemical change in the body, except if the devices are placed in the teeth, or to administer medicines, in which case they are in Class III.
- Directive 2003/12/EC introduced a derogation from this rule, reclassifying breast implants in Class III Directive 2005/50/EC introduced a derogation from this rule, reclassifying hip, knee and shoulder joint replacements in Class III.

Rule 9

Rule 9: Active therapeutic devices intended to administer or exchange energy.

Devices classified by this rule are mostly electrical equipment used in surgery such as lasers and surgical generators. In addition there are devices for specialised treatment such as radiation treatment. Another category consists of stimulation devices, although not all of them can be considered as delivering dangerous levels of energy considering the tissue involved.

Rule 9: All active therapeutic devices intended to administer or exchange energy are in Class IIa unless their characteristics are such that they may administer or exchange energy to and from the human body in a potentially hazardous way, taking account of the nature, the density and the site of application of the energy, in which case they are in Class IIb. All active devices intended to control or monitor the performance of active therapeutic devices in Class IIb or intended to influence directly the performance of such devices are in Class IIb.

Rule 10

Rule 10: Active devices for diagnosis. This primarily covers a whole range of widely used equipment in various fields, e.g. ultrasound diagnosis, capture of physiological signals and therapeutic and diagnostic radiology.

Rule 10: Active devices intended for diagnosis are in Class IIa:

- if they are intended to supply energy which will be absorbed by the human body, except for devices used to illuminate the patient's body, in the visible spectrum,
- if they are intended to image in vivo distribution of radiopharmaceuticals,
- if they are intended to allow direct diagnosis or monitoring of vital physiological processes,

unless they are specifically intended for monitoring of vital physiological parameters, where the nature of variations is such that it could result in immediate danger to the patient, for instance variations in cardiac performance, respiration, activity of CNS in which case they are in Class IIb.

Active devices intended to emit ionising radiation and intended for diagnostic and therapeutic interventional radiology including devices which control or monitor such devices, or which directly influence their performance, are in Class IIb.

Rule 11

Rule 11: Active devices intended to administer and/or remove medicines, body liquids or other substances to or from the body. This rule is intended to primarily cover drug delivery systems and anaesthesia equipment.

Rule 11: All active devices intended to administer and/or remove medicines, body liquids or other substances to or from the body are in Class IIa, unless this is done in a manner:
- that is potentially hazardous, taking account of the nature of the substances involved, of the part of the body concerned and of the mode of application, in which case they are in Class IIb.

Rule 12

Rule 12: All other active devices. This is a fall-back rule to cover all active devices not covered by the previous rules.

Rule 12: All other active devices are in Class I

Special Rules 12-18

Rule 13: Devices incorporating, as an integral part, a medicinal product or a human blood derivative (See MEDDEV. 2.1/3 for further guidance).
Rule 14: Devices used for contraception or prevention of sexually transmitted diseases.
Rule 15: Specific disinfecting, cleaning and rinsing devices.
Rule 16: Devices to record X-ray diagnostic images.
Rule 17: Devices utilising animal tissues or derivatives.
Rule 18: Blood bags.

CHAPTER 4
FDA REGULATION FOR MEDICAL DEVICES

Introduction

The FDA defines a medical device as "*A medical device is an instrument, apparatus, implement, machine, contrivance, implant or other similar or related article, including a component part, or accessory which is; Recognized in the official National Formulary, or the United States Pharmacopoeia, or any supplement to them, Intended for use in the cure, mitigation, treatment of disease, in man or other animals, or*
Intended to affect the structure or any function of the body of man or other animals, and which does not achieve any of it's primary intended purposes through chemical action within or on the body of man or other animals and which is not dependent upon being metabolized for the achievement of any of its primary intended purposes."

The FDA provides an online (www.ecfr.gov) electronic code of federal regulations (eCFR) which makes it very accessible to all manufacturers. The eCFR also provides the most up-to-date version of the code ensuring manufacturers comply with current requirements.

To understand the regulatory requirements of the FDA for medical devices, it is helpful to become familiar with the structure of the FDA Quality System (Part 820 Quality System Regulation). Below the title, chapter and subchapter for Medical devices are illustrated in the format per eCFR.

Title 21 → Chapter I → Subchapter H

TITLE 21—Food and Drugs

CHAPTER I—FOOD AND DRUG ADMINISTRATION, DEPARTMENT OF HEALTH AND HUMAN SERVICES (CONTINUED)

SUBCHAPTER H—MEDICAL DEVICES

Subchapter H-Medical Devices is then made up of Parts and subparts. Parts 800-898 refer to medical devices, with parts 900- Mammography Quality Standard Act and Part 1000-1050 Radiological health and so on as detailed below.

TITLE 21—Food and Drugs
SUBCHAPTER H—MEDICAL DEVICES

Part	Heading	Part	Heading
800	General	872	Dental Devices
801	Labeling	874	Ear, Nose, And Throat Devices
803	Medical Device Reporting	876	Gastroenterology-Urology Devices
806	Medical Devices; Reports Of Corrections And Removals	878	General And Plastic Surgery Devices
807	Establishment Registration And Device Listing For Manufacturers And Initial Importers Of Devices	880	General Hospital And Personal Use Devices
808	Exemptions From Federal Preemption Of State And Local Medical Device Requirements	882	Neurological Devices
809	In Vitro Diagnostic Products For Human Use	884	Obstetrical And Gynecological Devices
810	Medical Device Recall Authority	886	Ophthalmic Devices
812	Investigational Device Exemptions	888	Orthopedic Devices
813	[Reserved]	890	Physical Medicine Devices
814	Premarket Approval Of Medical Devices	892	Radiology Devices
820	Quality System Regulation	895	Banned Devices
821	Medical Device Tracking Requirements	898	Performance Standard For Electrode Lead Wires And Patient Cables
822	Postmarket Surveillance		
830	Unique Device Identification		
860	Medical Device Classification Procedures		
861	Procedures For Performance Standards Development		
862	Clinical Chemistry And Clinical Toxicology Devices		
864	Hematology And Pathology Devices		
866	Immunology And Microbiology Devices		
868	Anesthesiology Devices		
870	Cardiovascular Devices		

The section details the individual headings listed in Subchapter H (Medical Devices) along with a brief overview. Depending on product type and the product life cycle stage, reference to specific subparts may be warranted. However, Part 820-Quality system Regulation is most the most relevant to established manufacturers who wish to maintain the Quality system in a compliant fashion.

The below table outlines the content of Part 820- Quality System Regulation (Medical Devices). Subpart A through Subpart C are introductory in nature providing fundamental definitions and information. With regard to medical device manufacturers, Subpart C and Subpart G arguably require the greatest level of resources and expertise within an engineering and product environment.

An Overview of Subchapter H Medical Devices

Subpart A-General Provision

820.1 Scope
820.3 Definitions
820.5 Quality System

820.1 Scope

- o Part (a) of scope explains the "applicability" of CGMP requirements to medical devices.
- o The term "where appropriate" is detailed along with its meaning in terms of regulations. If a requirement is not appropriate, the manufacturer should have a justification documented to address non-implementation.
- o It also provides details in respect of (1) authority of the regulator (2) foreign manufacturers and their compliance and (3) exemptions also known as variances.

820.3 Definitions

- o This section defines the terms; Act, Complaint, Control, Design History File, Design Output, Device History file, Device master record, Establish, finished device, lot/batch, management with executive responsibility, manufacturer, rework, specification, remanufacturer and manufacturing material.
- o It also defines the following quality terms:

  - o **Quality** means the totality of features and characteristics that bear on the ability of a device to satisfy fitness-for-use, including safety and performance.

  - o **Quality audit** means a systematic, independent examination of a manufacturer's quality system that is performed at defined intervals and at sufficient frequency to determine whether both quality system activities and the results of such activities comply with quality system procedures, that these procedures are implemented effectively, and that these procedures are suitable to achieve quality system objectives.

  - o **Quality policy** means the overall intentions and direction of an organization with respect to quality, as established by management with executive responsibility.

- o **Quality system** means the organizational structure, responsibilities, procedures, processes, and resources for implementing quality management.

820.5 Quality System

This concise requirement states that:

- o Each manufacturer shall establish and maintain a quality system that is appropriate for the specific medical device(s) designed or manufactured, and that meets the requirements of this part.

Subpart B- Quality System Requirements

820.20 Management responsibility
820.22 Quality Audit
820.25 Personnel

820.20 Management responsibility

The first requirement of 820.20 is that a *Quality policy* is established. It is the management with executive responsibilities are responsible for the implementation of such Quality polices. Management must also ensure the *Organisation* is structured to ensure devices are designed and produced to meet regulatory requirements.

820.22 Quality Audit

This is also a direct and concise requirement that states:

"Each manufacturer shall establish procedures for quality audits and conduct such audits to assure that the quality system is in compliance with the established quality system requirements and to determine the effectiveness of the quality system. Quality audits shall be conducted by individuals who do not have direct responsibility for the matters being audited. Corrective action(s), including a re-audit of deficient matters, shall be taken when necessary. A report of the results of each quality audit, and re-audit(s) where taken, shall be made and such reports shall be reviewed by management having responsibility for the matters audited. The dates and results of quality audits and re-audits shall be documented"

820.25 Personnel

(a) *General.* Each manufacturer shall have sufficient personnel with the necessary education, background, training, and experience to assure that all activities required by this part are correctly performed.

(b) *Training.* Each manufacturer shall establish procedures for identifying training needs and ensure that all personnel are trained to adequately perform their assigned responsibilities. Training shall be documented.

(1) As part of their training, personnel shall be made aware of device defects which may occur from the improper performance of their specific jobs.

(2) Personnel who perform verification and validation activities shall be made aware of defects and errors that may be encountered as part of their job functions.

Subpart C- Design Controls

820.30 Design controls

Sections (a) through (y) provide definitions on common industry terms and Design controls such as complaint, component, design, device and so on. Starting a section (z) the regulation starts to delve into the validation and design requirements for medical devices.

(z)Validation means confirmation by examination and provision of objective evidence that the particular requirements for a specific intended use can be consistently fulfilled.

   (1) Process validation means establishing by objective evidence that a process consistently produces a result or product meeting its predetermined specifications.

   (2) Design validation means establishing by objective evidence that device specifications conform with user needs and intended use(s).

   (3) Verification means confirmation by examination and provision of objective evidence that specified requirements have been fulfilled.

Design validation: Each manufacturer shall establish and maintain procedures for validating the device design. Design validation shall be performed under defined operating conditions on initial production units, lots, or batches, or their equivalents. Design validation shall ensure that devices conform to defined user needs and intended uses and shall include testing of production units under actual or simulated use conditions. Design validation shall include software validation and risk analysis, where appropriate. The results of the design validation, including identification of the design, method(s), the date, and the individual(s) performing the validation, shall be documented in the DHF.

Design changes: Each manufacturer shall establish and maintain procedures for the identification, documentation, validation or where appropriate verification, review, and approval of design changes before their implementation.

Automated processes: When computers or automated data processing systems are used as part of production or the quality system, the manufacturer shall validate computer software for its intended use according to an established protocol. All software changes shall be validated before approval and issuance. These validation activities and results shall be documented.

Refer to Chapter 2 for additional information on principles of Design Control.

Subpart D-Document Controls

820.40 Document controls

"Each manufacturer shall establish and maintain procedures to control all documents that are required by this part. The procedures shall provide for the following:

(a) Document approval and distribution. Each manufacturer shall designate an individual(s) to review for adequacy and approve prior to issuance all documents established to meet the requirements of this part. The approval, including the date and signature of the individual(s) approving the document, shall be documented. Documents established to meet the requirements of this part shall be available at all locations for which they are designated, used, or otherwise necessary, and all obsolete documents shall be promptly removed from all points of use or otherwise prevented from unintended use.

(b) Document changes. Changes to documents shall be reviewed and approved by an individual(s) in the same function or organization that performed the original review and approval, unless specifically designated otherwise. Approved changes shall be communicated to the appropriate personnel in a timely manner. Each manufacturer shall maintain records of changes to documents. Change records shall include a description of the change, identification of the affected documents, the signature of the approving individual(s), the approval date, and when the change becomes effective."

Subpart E-Purchasing Controls

820.50 Purchasing controls

"Each manufacturer shall establish and maintain procedures to ensure that all purchased or otherwise received product and services conform to specified requirements.

(a) Evaluation of suppliers, contractors, and consultants. Each manufacturer shall establish and maintain the requirements, including quality requirements, that must be met by suppliers, contractors, and consultants. Each manufacturer shall:

(1) Evaluate and select potential suppliers, contractors, and consultants on the basis of their ability to meet specified requirements, including quality requirements. The evaluation shall be documented.

(2) Define the type and extent of control to be exercised over the product, services, suppliers, contractors, and consultants, based on the evaluation results.

(3) Establish and maintain records of acceptable suppliers, contractors, and consultants.

(b) Purchasing data. Each manufacturer shall establish and maintain data that clearly describe or reference the specified requirements, including quality requirements, for purchased or otherwise received product and services. Purchasing documents shall include, where possible, an agreement that the suppliers, contractors, and consultants agree to notify the manufacturer of changes in the product or service so that manufacturers may determine whether the changes may affect the quality of a finished device. Purchasing data shall be approved in accordance with §820.40."

Subpart F-Identification and Traceability

820.60   Identification
820.65   Traceability

820.60   Identification

"Each manufacturer shall establish and maintain procedures for identifying product during all stages of receipt, production, distribution, and installation to prevent mixups"

820.65   Traceability

"Each manufacturer of a device that is intended for surgical implant into the body or to support or sustain life and whose failure to perform when properly used in accordance with instructions for use provided in the labeling can be reasonably expected to result in a significant injury to the user shall establish and maintain procedures for identifying with a control number each unit, lot, or batch of finished devices and where appropriate components. The procedures shall facilitate corrective action. Such identification shall be documented in the DHR."

Subpart G- Production and Process Controls

820.70 Production and process controls

This section defines key elements of control that are necesssary within a manufacturing envirnment. Controls require systems to be in place to implement and monitor the application of controls, procedures and work practices:

"Production and process changes: Each manufacturer shall establish and maintain procedures for changes to a specification, method, process, or procedure. Such changes shall be verified or where appropriate validated according to §820.75, before implementation and these activities shall be documented. Changes shall be approved in accordance with §820.40.

Environmental control: Where environmental conditions could reasonably be expected to have an adverse effect on product quality, the manufacturer shall establish and maintain procedures to adequately control these environmental conditions. Environmental control system(s) shall be periodically inspected to verify that the system, including necessary equipment, is adequate and functioning properly. These activities shall be documented and reviewed.

Personnel: Each manufacturer shall establish and maintain requirements for the health, cleanliness, personal practices, and clothing of personnel if contact between such personnel and product or environment could reasonably be expected to have an adverse effect on product quality. The manufacturer shall ensure that maintenance and other personnel who are required to work temporarily under special environmental conditions are appropriately trained or supervised by a trained individual.

Contamination control: Each manufacturer shall establish and maintain procedures to prevent contamination of equipment or product by substances that could reasonably be expected to have an adverse effect on product quality.

Buildings: Buildings shall be of suitable design and contain sufficient space to perform necessary operations, prevent mixups, and assure orderly handling.

Equipment Each manufacturer shall ensure that all equipment used in the manufacturing process meets specified requirements and is appropriately designed, constructed, placed, and installed to facilitate maintenance, adjustment, cleaning, and use.

Maintenance schedule: Each manufacturer shall establish and maintain schedules for the adjustment, cleaning, and other maintenance of equipment to ensure that manufacturing specifications are met. Maintenance activities, including the date and individual(s) performing the maintenance activities, shall be documented.

Inspection: Each manufacturer shall conduct periodic inspections in accordance with established procedures to ensure adherence to applicable equipment maintenance schedules. The inspections, including the date and individual(s) conducting the inspections, shall be documented.

Adjustment: Each manufacturer shall ensure that any inherent limitations or allowable tolerances are visibly posted on or near equipment requiring periodic adjustments or are readily available to personnel performing these adjustments.

Manufacturing material: Where a manufacturing material could reasonably be expected to have an adverse effect on product quality, the manufacturer shall establish and maintain procedures for the use and removal of such manufacturing material to ensure that it is removed or limited to an amount that does not adversely affect the device's quality. The removal or reduction of such manufacturing material shall be documented.

Automated processes: When computers or automated data processing systems are used as part of production or the quality system, the manufacturer shall validate computer software for its intended use according to an established protocol. All software changes shall be validated before approval and issuance. These validation activities and results shall be documented.

820.72 Inspection, measuring and test equipment

Equipment must be fit for its *"intended purposes"* and produce *"valid"* results in a repeatable fashion. This section identifies the requirement of equipment to be traceable to a calibration standard with the appropriate evidence of calibration (calibration records).

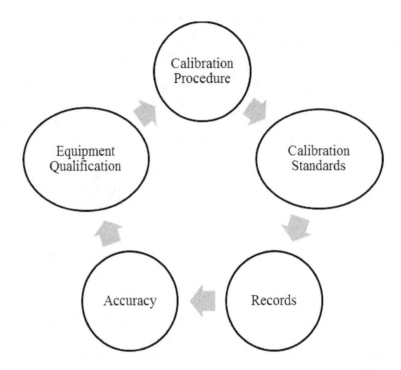

"Control of inspection, measuring, and test equipment: Each manufacturer shall ensure that all inspection, measuring, and test equipment, including mechanical, automated, or electronic inspection and test equipment, is suitable for its intended purposes and is capable of producing valid results. Each manufacturer shall establish and maintain procedures to ensure that equipment is routinely calibrated, inspected, checked, and maintained. The procedures shall include provisions for handling, preservation, and storage of equipment, so that its accuracy and fitness for use are maintained. These activities shall be documented.

Calibration: Calibration procedures shall include specific directions and limits for accuracy and precision. When accuracy and precision limits are not met, there shall be provisions for remedial action to re-establish the limits and to evaluate whether there was any adverse effect on the device's quality. These activities shall be documented.

Calibration standards: Calibration standards used for inspection, measuring, and test equipment shall be traceable to national or international standards. If national or international standards are not practical or available, the manufacturer shall use an independent reproducible standard. If no applicable standard exists, the manufacturer shall establish and maintain an in-house standard.

Calibration record: The equipment identification, calibration dates, the individual performing each calibration, and the next calibration date shall be documented. These records shall be displayed on or near each piece of equipment or shall be readily available to the personnel using such equipment and to the individuals responsible for calibrating the equipment."

Also relevant to calibrated test equipment is the following requirement as per Part 211.165 (e) *The accuracy, sensitivity, specificity, and reproducibility of test methods employed by the firm shall be established and documented. Such validation and documentation may be accomplished in accordance with 211.194(a)(2).*

820.75 Process Validation

(a) Where the results of a process cannot be fully verified by subsequent inspection and test, the process shall be validated with a high degree of assurance and approved according to established procedures. The validation activities and results, including the date and signature of the individual(s) approving the validation and where appropriate the major equipment validated, shall be documented.

(b) Each manufacturer shall establish and maintain procedures for monitoring and control of process parameters for validated processes to ensure that the specified requirements continue to be met.

   (1) Each manufacturer shall ensure that validated processes are performed by qualified individual(s)

   (2) For validated processes, the monitoring and control methods and data, the date performed, and, where appropriate, the individual(s) performing the process or the major equipment used shall be documented

(c) When changes or process deviations occur, the manufacturer shall review and evaluate the process and perform revalidation where appropriate. These activities shall be documented.

FDA Medical Device Guidance Section 4: Process Validation

The Quality System (QS) regulation defines process validation as establishing by objective evidence that a process consistently produces a result or product meeting its predetermined specifications [820.3(z)(1)].

The requirement for process validation appears in section 820.75 of the Quality System (QS) regulation. The goal of a quality system is to consistently produce products that are fit for their intended use. Process validation is a key element in assuring that these principles and goals are met.

Processes are developed according to the design controls in 820.30 and validated according to 820.75. The process specifications, hereafter called parameters, are derived from the specifications for the device, component or other entity to be produced by the process.

The parameters are documented in the device master record per 820.30, 820.40 and 820.181. The process is developed such that the required parameters are achieved. To ensure that the output of the process will consistently meet the required parameters during routine production, the process is validated.

The basic principles for validation are suggested as follows:

- *"Establish that the process equipment has the capability of operating within required parameters;*
- *Demonstrate that controlling, monitoring, and/or measuring equipment and instrumentation are capable of operating within the parameters prescribed for the process equipment;*
- *Perform replicate cycles (runs) representing the required operational range of the equipment to demonstrate that the processes have been operated within the prescribed parameters for the process and that the output or product consistently meets predetermined specifications for quality and function; and*
- *Monitor the validated process during routine operation. As needed, requalify and recertify the equipment."*

Subpart H- Acceptance Activities

820.80 Receiving, in-process and finished device acceptance

820.86 Acceptance status

820.80 Receiving, in-process and finished device acceptance

(a) General. Each manufacturer shall establish and maintain procedures for acceptance activities. Acceptance activities include inspections, tests, or other verification activities.

(b) Receiving acceptance activities. Each manufacturer shall establish and maintain procedures for acceptance of incoming product. Incoming product shall be inspected, tested, or otherwise verified as conforming to specified requirements. Acceptance or rejection shall be documented.

(c) In-process acceptance activities. Each manufacturer shall establish and maintain acceptance procedures, where appropriate, to ensure that specified requirements for in-process product are met. Such procedures shall ensure that in-process product is controlled until the required inspection and tests or other verification activities have been completed, or necessary approvals are received, and are documented.

820.86 Acceptance status

"Each manufacturer shall identify by suitable means the acceptance status of product, to indicate the conformance or nonconformance of product with acceptance criteria. The identification of acceptance status shall be maintained throughout manufacturing, packaging, labeling, installation, and servicing of the product to ensure that only product which has passed the required acceptance activities is distributed, used, or installed"

In simple terms, the acceptance status of a product or component is determined by inspection or testing. This may be done via a sample based approach. Conformance or non-conformance of products needs to be determined with reference to an approved specification or standard. In order to satisfy this requirement, product must then be identified as conforming or not. This may be achieved by using lot/batch numbers or other means of identifying product.

Subpart-I Non-conforming Product

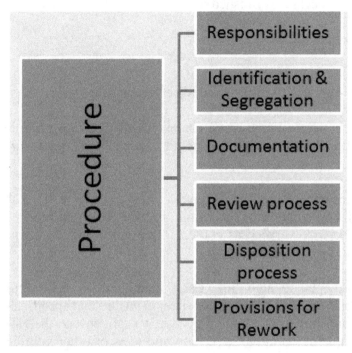

The requirements for Non-conforming products are principally driven by site or company procedure. The procedure should address the above key points and provide sufficient information to allow non-conforming product to be effectively identified and managed.

"(a) Control of nonconforming product. Each manufacturer shall establish and maintain procedures to control product that does not conform to specified requirements. The procedures shall address the identification, documentation, evaluation, segregation, and disposition of nonconforming product. The evaluation of non-conformance shall include a determination of the need for an investigation and notification of the persons or organizations responsible for the non-conformance. The evaluation and any investigation shall be documented.

(b) Non-conformity review and disposition. (1) Each manufacturer shall establish and maintain procedures that define the responsibility for review and the authority for the disposition of nonconforming product. The procedures shall set forth the review and disposition process. Disposition of nonconforming product shall be documented. Documentation shall include the justification for use of nonconforming product and the signature of the individual(s) authorizing the use.

(2) Each manufacturer shall establish and maintain procedures for rework, to include retesting and re-evaluation of the nonconforming product after rework, to ensure that the product meets its current approved specifications. Rework and re-evaluation activities, including a determination of any adverse effect from the rework upon the product, shall be documented in the DHR."

Subpart J-Corrective and Preventive Action

820.100 Corrective and preventive action

The below process outlines the steps and key elements of corrective and preventive action as prescribed by 820.100

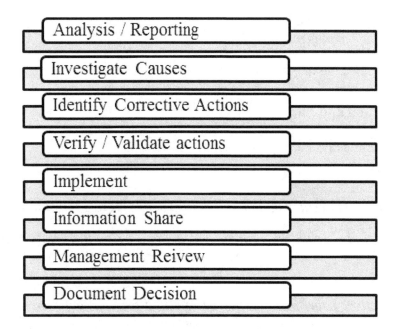

The text of 820.10 states the following:

(a) Each manufacturer shall establish and maintain procedures for implementing corrective and preventive action. The procedures shall include requirements for:

(1) Analyzing processes, work operations, concessions, quality audit reports, quality records, service records, complaints, returned product, and other sources of quality data to identify existing and potential causes of nonconforming product, or other quality problems. Appropriate statistical methodology shall be employed where necessary to detect recurring quality problems;

(2) Investigating the cause of nonconformities relating to product, processes, and the quality system;

(3) Identifying the action(s) needed to correct and prevent recurrence of nonconforming product and other quality problems;

(4) Verifying or validating the corrective and preventive action to ensure that such action is effective and does not adversely affect the finished device;

(5) Implementing and recording changes in methods and procedures needed to correct and prevent identified quality problems;

(6) Ensuring that information related to quality problems or nonconforming product is disseminated to those directly responsible for assuring the quality of such product or the prevention of such problems; and

(7) Submitting relevant information on identified quality problems, as well as corrective and preventive actions, for management review.

(b) All activities required under this section, and their results, shall be documented"

Subpart K—Labeling and Packaging Control

820.12 Device Labeling and Packaging Control

"Each manufacturer shall establish and maintain procedures to control labeling activities.

(a) Label integrity. Labels shall be printed and applied so as to remain legible and affixed during the customary conditions of processing, storage, handling, distribution, and where appropriate use.

(b) Labeling inspection. Labeling shall not be released for storage or use until a designated individual(s) has examined the labeling for accuracy including, where applicable, the correct unique device identifier (UDI) or universal product code (UPC), expiration date, control number, storage instructions, handling instructions, and any additional processing instructions. The release, including the date and signature of the individual(s) performing the examination, shall be documented in the DHR.

(c) Labeling storage. Each manufacturer shall store labeling in a manner that provides proper identification and is designed to prevent mixups.

(d) Labeling operations. Each manufacturer shall control labeling and packaging operations to prevent labeling mixups. The label and labeling used for each production unit, lot, or batch shall be documented in the DHR.

(e) Control number. Where a control number is required by §820.65, that control number shall be on or shall accompany the device through distribution."

820.13 Device packaging

"Each manufacturer shall ensure that device packaging and shipping containers are designed and constructed to protect the device from alteration or damage during the customary conditions of processing, storage, handling, and distribution."

CHAPTER 5

EUROPEAN REGULATION FOR MEDICAL DEVICES

Directives

90/385/ECC– The Active Implantable Medical Devices Directive (AIMDI)
93/42/ECC – The Medical Devices Directive (MDD)
98/79/EEC – In Vitro Diagnostic MDD (IVDMDD)

What are MEDDEVs?

The MEDDEVs are guidance documents that aim to promote a common approach to be followed by manufacturers and Notified Bodies (e.g. FDA, MHRA etc.) that are involved in conformity assessment procedures for products.

- The MEDDEVs are drafted by European authorities charged with safeguarding public health in conjunction with all stakeholders; industry associations, health professionals associations, Notified Bodies and European Standardisation Organisations.

- MEDDEVs are carefully drafted through a consultation process with all interested parties and are subject to a regular updating process

- It is important to understand that the MEDDEV guidelines are not legally binding. However, it is expected and typically the standard practice to follow guidelines.

In addition, to MEDDEVs, consensus statements and informative documents aim to ensure uniform application of directives within the EU. From April 2017 all guidance and implementing measures under the current Directives are to be reviewed over the next few years in the light of the texts of the 2 new Regulations.

Below is a complete list of all Guidance Meddevs published titles:

Reference/Application	Title
2.1 Scope, filed of application, definition	**MEDDEV 2.1/1** Definitions of "medical devices", "accessory" and "manufacturer" **April 1994**
	MEDDEV 2.1/2 rev.2 Field of application of directive "active implantable medical devices" **April 1994**

	MEDDEV 2.1/2.1 Treatment of Computers Used to Program Implantable Pulse Generators **February 1998**
	MEDDEV 2.1/3 rev.3 Borderline products, drug-delivery products and medical devices incorporating, as integral part, an ancillary medicinal substance or an ancillary human blood derivative **December 2009**
	MEDDEV 2.1/4 Interface with other directives – Medical devices/directive 89/336/EEC relating to electromagnetic compatibility and directive 89/686/EEC relating to personal protective equipment **March 1994** For the relation between the MDD and directive 89/686/EEC concerning personal protective equipment, please see the Commission services **interpretative document of 21 August 2009**
	MEDDEV 2.1/5 Medical devices with a measuring function **June 1998**
	MEDDEV 2.1/6 Qualification and Classification of stand alone software **July 2016**

Reference/Application	Title
2.2 Essential requirements	**MEDDEV 2.2/1 rev.1** EMC requirements **February 1998**
	MEDDEV 2.2/3 rev.3 "Use by"-date **June 1998**
	MEDDEV 2.2/4 Conformity assessment of IN VITRO Fertilisation (IVF) and Assisted Reproduction Technologies (ART) products **January 2012**

Reference/Application	Title
2.4 Classification of MD	**MEDDEV 2.4/1 rev.9** Classification of medical devices **June 2010**
2.5 Conformity assessment procedure	Quality assurance. Regulatory auditing of quality systems of medical device manufacturers **(See document in the GHTF-Global Harmonization Task Force)**
	MEDDEV 2.5/3 rev.2 Subcontracting quality systems related

	June 1998
	MEDDEV 2.5/5 rev.3 Translation procedure **February 1998**
	MEDDEV 2.5/6 rev.1 Homogenous batches (verification of manufacturers' products) **February 1998**

Reference/Application	Title
	Conformity assessment for particular groups of products
2.5 Conformity Assessment procedure	**MEDDEV 2.5/7 rev.1** Conformity assessment of breast implants **July 1998**
	MEDDEV 2.5/9 rev.1 Evaluation of medical devices incorporating products containing natural rubber latex **February 2004**
	MEDDEV 2.5/10 Guideline for Authorised Representatives **January 2012**

Reference/Application	Title
2.7 **Clinical investigation, clinical evaluation**	**MEDDEV 2.7/1 rev.4** Clinical evaluation: Guide for manufacturers and notified bodies **June 2016** **Appendix 1: Clinical evaluation on coronary stents December 2008**
	MEDDEV 2.7/2 rev. 2 Guidelines for Competent Authorities for making a validation/assessment of a clinical investigation application under directives 90/385/EEC and 93/42/EC **September 2015**
	MEDDEV 2.7/3 rev. 3 Clinical investigations: serious adverse reporting under directives 90/385/EEC and 93/42/EC - SAE reporting form **May 2015** **The new SAE reporting form will be taken in use 1 September 2016 at the latest.**
	MEDDEV 2.7/4 Guidelines on Clinical investigations: a guide for manufacturers and notified bodies **December 2010**

Reference/Application	Title
2.10 Notified bodies	**MEDDEV 2.10/2 rev.1** (105 kB) Designation and monitoring of Notified Bodies within the framework of EC Directives on Medical devices **Annex 1** (119 kB), **Annex 2** (14 kB), **Annex 3** (16 kB), **Annex 4** (26 kB) **April 2001**

Reference/Application	Title
2.12 **Market surveillance**	**MEDDEV 2.12/1 rev.8** (763 kB) Guidelines on a Medical Devices Vigilance System **January 2013**

Reference/Application	Title
2.13 Transitional period	**MEDDEV 2.13 rev.1** Commission communication on the application of transitional provision of Directive 93/42/EEC relating to medical devices (OJ 98/C 242/05) **August 1998**

Reference/Application	Title
2.14 IVD	**MEDDEV 2.14/1 rev.2** (76 kB) Borderline and Classification issues. A guide for manufacturers and notified bodies **January 2012**
	MEDDEV 2.14/2 rev.1 (64 kB) Research Use Only products **February 2004**
	MEDDEV 2.14/3 rev.1 (80 kB) Supply of Instructions For Use (IFU) and other information for In-vitro Diagnostic (IVD)Medical Devices **January 2007**
	Form for the registration of manufacturers and devices **In Vitro Diagnostic Medical Device** **Directive, Article 10** (213 kB) **January 2007**
	MEDDEV 2.14/4 (114 kB) CE marking of blood based in vitro diagnostic medical devices for vCJD based on detection of abnormal PrP

January 2012

Reference/Application	Title
2.15 **Other guidance**	**MEDDEV 2.15 rev.3** (32 kB) Committees/Working Groups contributing to the implementation of the Medical Device Directives **December 2008**

Reference/Application	Title
2.10 Notified bodies	**MEDDEV 2.10/2 rev.1** (105 kB) Designation and monitoring of Notified Bodies within the framework of EC Directives on Medical devices **Annex 1** (119 kB), **Annex 2** (14 kB), **Annex 3** (16 kB), **Annex 4** (26 kB) **April 2001**

These documents can be accessed via the internet web address - http://ec.europa.eu/growth/sectors/medical-devices/guidance/#meddevs

CHAPTER 6

MEDICAL SOFTWARE AND APPS

Introduction

Software applications also known as "apps" have become a mainstream phenomenon for mobile phones and tablets and other personal electronic devices. Apps have crossed over into the health and fitness sector that allow personal devices to track and report physical activity, sleep and provide health tips. Furthermore medical devices also offer increased interaction with "apps" allowing real-time analysis of physiological data.

How to determine if a software app is a medical device?

In simple terms, any software app that provides a diagnostic function in order to determine disease or a medical condition is likely to fall under the definition of a medical device. Examples include:

- Apps that calculate medicine doses a patient is to take
- Apps that identify or inform you that you have a particular medical condition or disease
- Apps provide a risk based assessment

CE marking of Devices

When an app developer applies a 'CE mark' they are claiming that the app is fit for the purpose (aka the intended purpose) and it is acceptably safe to use. The CE mark should be visible on the app when you are looking at it in the app store, the 'landing' page or on the app developer's product website or information page. The manufacturer has a duty to provide clear information that describes what the app can be used for and how to use it.

Consumers should exercise caution when purchasing apps from unknown sources. Product not CE marked or products not assessed for safety pose a potential risk when used. Any medical device app that does not have a CE mark evident from literature, manufacturers information or interface should be reported to the relevant competent authority.

Personal data and apps

Many apps have the ability to capture and record physiological parameters such as heart rate, sleep patterns and activity. Many also support the input of additional data such as as persons weight and physical attributes. This baseline can be further supplemented with

It is very important that you have read the small print to understand what personal data you may have agreed to share with the developer by signing up to the app and how they might store or use your data or share your information with third parties.

This includes information about you such as your name, address, date of birth and information about your health.

General Guidance on Use

Once you are sure the app is right for you and it is CE marked then you should follow the instructions carefully.

Be honest with the information you put into the app. If you enter wrong information about yourself, the app may not give you the right result. Ensure that you always update the app to the newest compatible version.

After using

If you are in doubt about the information that the app has given you or you are concerned about your health then you should consult a healthcare professional (a pharmacist, health visitor, practice nurse or GP) If you have any problems with the app not working as stated e.g.

• If the instructions aren't clear or the app is difficult to use
• If the app isn't giving you the results that you expected
• If you have concerns over the safety of the app or the information that it provides

European Requirements –Stand-alone Software

This guideline on the qualification and classification of stand-alone software was drafted by the European Commission after consultation of the competent authorities, commission services, industry and notified bodies

MEDDEV 2.1/6 rev. 1: Qualification and classification of stand-alone software

A stand-alone software must meet the following criteria in order to be classified as a medical device:

      o   it has to be a computer program

o the software has to have a different purpose than mere storage, archival, lossless compression, communication or simple search

o the software has to be for the benefit of individual patients

o the software has to have an intended purpose listed in Article 1(2)a) of Directive 93/42/EEC.
(In Germany, Article 1(2)a) of Directive 93/42/EEC has been implemented as national law in Section 3 number 1 MPG.)

FDA Requirements

Food and Drug Administration FDA: "Mobile Medical Applications -Guidance for Industry and Food and Drug Administration Staff", February 2015

Introduction

Issued in 2015, the FDA provided non-binding guidance on "Mobile Medical Applications". The aim of the guidance is to inform industry on how the FDA intends to apply its regulatory authorities to select software applications intended for use on mobile platform/mobile apps.

The guidance also states that although some mobile apps may meet the definition of a medical device, if they propose a lower risk to the public FDA intends to exercise enforcement discretion over these devices.

As mobile platforms become more user friendly, computationally powerful, and readily available, innovators have begun to develop mobile apps of increasing complexity to leverage the portability mobile platforms can offer.

Some of these new mobile apps are specifically targeted to assisting individuals in their own health and wellness management. Other mobile apps are targeted to healthcare providers as tools to improve and facilitate the delivery of patient care.

These software devices include products that feature one or more software components, parts, or accessories (such as electrocardiographic (ECG) systems used to monitor cardiac rhythms), as well as devices that are composed solely of software (such as laboratory information management systems).

On February 15, 2011, the FDA issued a regulation down classifying certain computer- or software-based devices intended to be used for the electronic transfer, storage, display, and/or format conversion of medical device data – called Medical Device Data Systems (MDDSs) – from Class III (high-risk) to Class I (low-risk).2 The FDA has previously clarified that when stand-alone software is used to analyze medical device data, it has traditionally been regulated as an accessory to a medical device3 or as medical device software.

As is the case with traditional medical devices, certain mobile medical apps can pose potential risks to public health. Moreover, certain mobile medical apps may pose risks that are unique to the characteristics of the platform on which the mobile medical app is run interpretation of radiological images on a mobile device could be adversely affected by the smaller screen size, lower contrast ratio, and uncontrolled ambient light of the mobile platform.

FDA intends to take these risks into account in assessing the appropriate regulatory oversight for these products. This guidance clarifies and outlines the FDA's current thinking.

The Agency will continue to evaluate the potential impact these technologies might have on improving health care, reducing potential medical mistakes, and protecting patients.

Definitions

Mobile Platform: For purposes of this guidance, "mobile platforms" are defined as commercial off-the-shelf (COTS) computing platforms, with or without wireless connectivity, that are handheld in nature. Examples of these mobile platforms include mobile computers such as smart phones, tablet computers, or other portable computers.

Mobile Application (Mobile App): For purposes of this guidance, a mobile application or "mobile app" is defined as a software application that can be executed (run) on a mobile platform (i.e., a handheld commercial off-the shelf computing platform, with or without wireless connectivity), or a web-based software application that is tailored to a mobile platform but is executed on a server.

Mobile Medical Application (Mobile Medical App): For purposes of this guidance, a "mobile medical app" is a mobile app that meets the definition of device in section 201(h) of the Federal Food, Drug, and Cosmetic Act (FD&C Act) - 7 - 4 ; and either is intended:

· to be used as an accessory to a regulated medical device; or
to transform a mobile platform into a regulated medical device.

Mobile Medical App: the FDA defines a "mobile medical app manufacturer" is any person or entity that manufactures mobile medical apps in accordance with the definitions of manufacturer in 21 CFR Parts 803, 806, 807, and 820.

They may include companies that initiates specifications, designs, labels, or creates a software system or application for a regulated medical device in whole or from multiple software components.

BfArM Germany

Guidance from the Federal Institute for Drugs and Medical Devices (BfArM), Germany

Differentiation between apps and medical or other devices as well as on the subsequent risk classification according to the MPG

BfArM as with other competent Authorities provides guidance on differentiation between:

(1) apps (in general: stand-alone software, not incorporated into a medical device, e.g. as control software) and

(2) medical devices.

In similar fashion, any this guidance is informative and non- binding. Qualification and classification needs to determine the intended purpose of the software and its classification must is the responsibility of the manufacturer.

- Differentiation/Qualification
- Risk Classification
- Examples for Differerientation/qualification
- Further Guidance
- European Commission
- Other Authorities
- Committees

Differentiation and Qualification

The "intended purpose" is the use for which the medical device is intended according to the manufacturer's information, marketing, labelling and instructions for use (IFU).

Thus, not only the explicitly described intended purpose is relevant e.g. for an authority decision on qualification as a medical device, but also the instructions for use and the promotional materials (e.g. website, information in App Store) regarding the specific product.

BfArM guidance also points out that Stand alone software such as smartphone apps can indeed be classified as a medical device. However the product must be intended by the manufacturer to be used for humans with a minimum of at least one of the criteria below fufilled:

- diagnosis, prevention, monitoring, treatment or alleviation of disease,

- diagnosis, monitoring, treatment, alleviation or compensation of injuries or handicaps,

- investigation, replacement or modification of the anatomy or of a physiological process,

- control of conception.

Essentially, the above criteria is a summary of the European regulations pertaining to medical devices.

As opposed to mere provision of knowledge, e.g. in a paper or electronic book (no medical device), any type of interference with data or information by the stand alone software is indicative of a classification as a medical device.

Possible indicative terms in connection with the intended purpose of corresponding functions can be e.g.: alarm, analyse, calculate, detect, diagnose, interpret, convert, measure, control, monitor, amplify.

Indicative functions for classification as a medical device can be among the following:

- decision support or decision making software e.g. with regard to therapeutic measures

- calculation e.g. of dosing of medicines (as opposed to mere reproduction of a table from which users can deduce the dosage themselves)

- monitoring patients and collecting data e.g. by measurements if the results thereof have an influence on diagnosis or therapy.

Pure data storage, archiving, lossless compression, communication or simple search functions do not result in classification as a medical device.

Like all other medical devices from own production, software applications from own production are medical devices and thus must fulfil the basic requirements of Council Directive 93/42/EEC.

Risk Classification

With the exception of in vitro diagnostic medical devices and active implantable medical devices, medical devices are allocated to risk classes that are mainly based on the potential damage that can be caused by an error/malfunction of the medical device.

These risk classes range from Class I (low risk) and IIa and IIb to Class III (high risk). Class I products are additionally subdivided according to whether they require sterilisation (Is) or include a measuring function (Im) which is relevant for the further conformity assessment procedure.

The classification is based on the rules laid down in Annex IX of Council Directive 93/42/EEC. The following rules are most suitable for the classification of stand alone software:

Rule 9

"All active therapeutic devices intended to administer or exchange energy are in Class IIa unless their characteristics are such that they may administer or exchange energy to or from the human body in a potentially hazardous way, taking account of the nature, the density and site of application of the energy, in which case they are in Class IIb. All active devices intended to control or monitor the performance of active therapeutic devices in Class IIb, or intended directly to influence the performance of such devices are in Class IIb."

Rule 10

"Active devices intended for diagnosis are in Class IIa,

- if they are intended to supply energy which will be absorbed by the human body, except for devices used to illuminate the patient's body, in the visible spectrum;

- if they are intended to image in vivo distribution of radiopharmaceuticals;

- if they are intended to allow direct diagnosis or monitoring of vital physiological processes, unless they are specifically intended for monitoring of vital physiological parameters, where the nature of variations is such that it could result in immediate danger to the patient, for instance variations in cardiac performance, respiration, activity of CNS in which case they are in Class IIb.

- Active devices intended to emit ionizing radiation and intended for diagnostic and therapeutic interventional radiology including devices which control or monitor such devices, or which directly influence their performance, are in Class IIb."

Rule 12

"All other active devices are in Class I."

Rule 14

"All devices used for contraception or the prevention of the transmission of sexually transmitted diseases are in Class IIb, ..."

The following definitions in accordance with Annex IX Section I No. 1 of Council Directive 93/42/EEC are to be observed:

- **Stand alone software**

  Stand alone software is considered to be an active medical device.

- **Active therapeutical device**

  "Any active medical device, whether used alone or in combination with other medical devices, to support, modify, replace or restore biological functions or structures with a view to treatment or alleviation of an illness, injury or handicap."

- **Active device for diagnosis**

  "Any active medical device, whether used alone or in combination with other medical devices, to supply information for detecting, diagnosing, monitoring or treating physiological conditions, states of health, illnesses or congenital deformities."

The afore-mentioned rules show that e.g. medical apps on smartphones and tablets will mostly be classified in risk Class I in accordance with Rule 12.

If the medical devices are intended for diagnosis or monitoring of vital functions (e.g. cardiac functions), Classes IIa or IIb can also be considered.

Depending on the risk class there are different requirements for conducting a conformity assessment procedure as the prerequisite for affixing the CE marking and for correct marketing within the European Economic Area.

Thus, the manufacturer can perform a conformity assessment e.g. for Class I devices without involvement of a notified body; for all other risk classes (also in the case of Class I devices that require sterilisation or include a measuring function) it is mandatory to involve a notified body.

If a stand alone software or app is placed on the market as a medical device it is subject to the same regulations as all other medical devices.

Examples for Qualification/differentiation

Decision supporting software

In general, software is usually considered a medical device when it is used for healthcare, if e.g. medical knowledge databases and algorithms are combined with patient-specific data and the software is intended to give healthcare professionals recommendations on diagnosis, prognosis, monitoring or treatment of an individual patient.

Software systems

If a software consists of several modules it is the manufacturer's responsibility whether he wants the modules as a whole to be qualified and classified or each module individually. If the entire system is qualified and if it consists both of software with and without the properties of a medical device, the system is subject to medical device legislation.

Telemedical software

In telemedicine the physician observes and assesses the patients' medical data using telecommunication technologies - e.g. via the internet. Patient and physician can be at different locations.

Depending on the intended purpose, communication systems for telemedicine can either be non-medical devices (purely for transfer of data) or a combination of non-medical devices and medical devices (e.g. in order to support diagnoses).

Hospital information systems (HIS)

Hospital information systems that support patient management are generally not medical devices, especially if they have the following intended purpose:

- o collection of data for patient admission
- o administration of general patient data

- scheduling of appointments
- insurance and billing functions

However, hospital information systems can be combined with other modules that could be medical devices.

Picture Archiving and Communication System (PACS)

For example, if the manufacturer of the PACS software specifies in the intended purpose that the software is only meant for storage or archiving of pictures and not for diagnosing, this would indicate that it is not a medical device. However, if the manufacturer intends the PACS software for controlling a medical device or to have an influence on its use or to allow a direct diagnosis, this would support its classification as a medical device.

Stand alone software or apps that are **not** medical devices

Operating system software:
Operating system software (e.g. Windows, Linux) is neither a medical device nor is it an accessory to a medical device.

Software for general purposes

Software for general purposes is not a medical device even if it is used in connection with healthcare.

Software or apps as health or fitness products
When differentiating medical devices e.g. from health or fitness products, the decisive issue is whether they are intended for medical or non-medical purposes. This is defined by the manufacturer of the product. Software or apps merely intended for sporting activities, fitness, well-being or nutritional aims without a medical purpose claimed by the manufacturer are generally not medical devices

Medicines and Healthcare products Regulatory Agency, MHRA

Introduction

The Medicines and Healthcare products Regulatory Agency (MHRA) is an agency of the Department of Health in the UK which is responsible for ensuring that medicines and medical devices work and are acceptably safe.

Formed in 2003 with the merger of the Medicines Control Agency (MCA) and the Medical Devices Agency (MDA). In April 2013, it merged with the National Institute for Biological Standards and Control (NIBSC) and as the MHRA. The MHRA has released guidance on Medical Device stand-alone software including apps (Aug 2014). This guidance should be used in addition to MEDDEV 2.1/6.

Medicines & Healthcare products Regulatory Agency (MHRA): Guidance - Medical device stand-alone software including Apps, August 2014

Medical device stand-alone software including apps (including IVDMDs)

As well as medical device apps becoming a growth area in healthcare management in hospital and in the community settings, the role of apps used as part of fitness regimes and for social care situations is also expanding.

However, in the UK and throughout Europe, standalone software and apps that meet the definition of a medical device are still required to be CE marked in line with the EU medical device directives in order to ensure they are regulated and acceptably safe to use and also perform in the way the manufacturer/ developer intends them to.

Health related apps and software that are not medical devices can be extremely useful but fall outside the scope of the MHRA.

But how do developers and users of this software decide whether apps qualify as medical devices and which are for health and fitness purposes?

When apps are not medical devices

Those apps that are not medical devices may be considered to be mHealth products. Work is ongoing at European level to determine a suitable legal framework.

The Concept of Mobile Health (mHealth)

Mobile health (hereafter "mHealth") covers *"medical and public health practice supported by mobile devices, such as mobile phones, patient monitoring devices, personal digital assistants (PDAs), and other wireless devices"*

It also includes applications (hereafter "apps") such as lifestyle and wellbeing apps[2] that may connect to medical devices or sensors (e.g. bracelets or watches) as well as personal guidance systems, health information and medication reminders provided by sms and telemedicine provided wirelessly.

mHealth is an emerging and rapidly developing field which has the potential to play a part in the transformation of healthcare and increase its quality and efficiency.

mHealth solutions cover various technological solutions, that among others measure vital signs such as heart rate, blood glucose level, blood pressure, body temperature and brain activities. Prominent examples of apps are communication, information and motivation tools, such as medication reminders or tools offering fitness and dietary recommendations. The expanding spread of smartphones as well as 3G and 4G networks has boosted the use of mobile apps offering healthcare services. The availability of satellite navigation technologies in mobile devices provides the possibility to improve the safety and autonomy of patients. Through sensors and mobile apps, mHealth allows the collection of considerable medical, physiological, lifestyle, daily activity and environmental data. This could serve as a basis for evidence-driven care practice and research activities, while facilitating patients' access to their health information anywhere and at any time.

mHealth could also support the delivery of high-quality healthcare, and enable more accurate diagnosis and treatment. It can support healthcare professionals in treating patients more efficiently as mobile apps can encourage adherence to a healthy lifestyle, resulting in more personalised medication and treatment.

It can contribute to the empowerment of patients as they could manage their health more actively, living more independent lives in their own home environment thanks to self-assessment or remote monitoring solutions and monitoring of environmental factors such as changes in air quality that might influence medical conditions. In this respect, mHealth is not intended to replace healthcare professionals who remain central to providing healthcare but rather is considered to be a supportive tool for the management and provision of healthcare.

Benefits and Issues with mHealth

Benefits
- Disease Prevention
- More Efficient Healthcare
- Empowers Patients
- Quality of Life
- Reduce Healthcare costs

Issues
- Data Protection
- Liability
- Interoperability
- App Certification
- Errobeous Data

CHAPTER 7

TEST METHODS

Introduction

This guidebook covers the design, execution and analysis of test method validation for medical devices. Test method validation involves the formal documentation of a test method used to capture and analyse data or information. The reason test methods need to be validated is to confirm that they are suitable and fit for the intended purpose. Secondly, and of equal importance is the need to verify that the test method performs to an acceptable level and is reliable and trustworthy over time. After all, test methods are used to assess product outputs such as dimensions, material strength and product functions. Getting this wrong will lead nowhere very quickly, so it is important to have confidence in the results of testing.

Validation studies must demonstrate method capabilities in the testing environment. As a result, validation studies allow the formal documentation of the ruggedness of the test method in real-use conditions (i.e. demonstrating that the precision and accuracy limits are met with different technicians, different production batches and variable test equipment, etc.).

Examples of Test Method Validations

Example 1

A packaging company has a seal strength on the lid of a package. It wants to put in place a test method to test the seal strength of the package. This scenario would call for a test method validation.

Example 2

A medical device incorporates the use of a spring that is used to actuate a valve. The manufacturer of the device wants to develop a test method that examines the tensile strength of the spring on an ongoing basis. This scenario would also call for a test method validation.

Example 3

A contact lens manufacturer uses an optical comparator to measure the diameter of contact lenses during manufacture. The manufacturer must develop and validate a test method to facilitate the measuring of contact lenses.

What is test method validation?

Test method validation is the documented process of ensuring a test method is suitable for its intended use.

The intended use of any system is normally documented and described in a User Requirements Specification. Test method validation involves establishing the performance characteristics and limitations of a method and the identification of influences which may change those characteristics.

Why should TMV be performed?

TMV is an important element of quality control. Without validation there can be no assurance that the test results will be reliable and fit for the purpose. In some fields, validation of methods is a regulatory requirement. Generally, any method used to produce data in support of regulatory (e.g., FDA) filings or the manufacture of devices for human use should be validated.

All are candidates for validation, though the process for each can vary. Most test methods exist as validated standards, methods developed by technical standard organizations (ANSI, ASTM, ISO…) to establish uniform methods and procedures for testing. But standard methods do not always fit the requirements of the tests to be performed.

When should methods be validated?

The risk associated with products an output (dimensions, features, chemical requirements etc.) often dictates the validation activity based on the potential level of patient harm weighed against the business risk of not performing the activities.

The device risk index or harm classification dictates the minimum level of statistical confidence required. Higher risk requires more rigorous testing and higher levels of statistical confidence. In most cases, TMV is not mandated in the medical device industry (except ISO 11607). But demonstrating the safety and effectiveness of a device is difficult to do if the methods for establishing these parameters are not shown to be appropriate and reliable. Test Method Validation may be required for:

- A new method is developed
- A revision to established methods
- Methods that are moved or transferred

Changes Requiring Re-Validation

Take the case where a standard test method is established and in operation. However, a change to the system software is required. This type of change could impact the measured output. Therefore the change needs to be considered for re-validation.

Any other changes to the test procedure such as a change in handling of test specimens or the change, addition, removal or modification of equipment including fixturing can impact the measured output.

It is important to note that validation of a test method is not required on each individual piece of equipment or fixturing, once replicate equipment or fixturing is assessed during the validation study.

Some examples of changes not necessarily requiring any re-validation or change to a validation report etc. include:

- Clerical corrections to the test method that do not change the method or affect the measurement of the output.

- Removing of referenced supplies that do not impact test output, for example lint or cleaning agents.

- Movement of equipment does normally not merit re-validation of the test method, but a limited equipment qualification may be required.

Test method validations should be product and site specific. This means the site and product should be clearly defined in the scope of the test method validation documents. Before an already existing validated test method can be used with a new product or at a new site, the suitability of the existing test method must be documented.

The Code of Federal Regulations (CFR) Title 21 Part 820: Quality System Regulation (QSR) 21 does not clearly call out requirements on method validation. It does not actually mentions the words "method" and "validation" side by side. However, many warning letters have been issued to manufacturing on the subject since at least 2005. Method validation also protects the manufacturer from allowing defective product to circumvent inspection methods if not fit for purpose.

Regulating guidelines from a variety of sources covered in the sections below. The discussion, as it relates to method validation, is somewhat circuitous for medical devices. As stated previously, this is caused by the absence of the phrase method validation in FDA QSR documents. For this reason, some basic treatment relating to process validation is covered below even though this topic is covered in detail in a separate chapter especially because the actual CFR definitions are general enough to lump methods into the category of a process if a CDRH auditor sees fit to do so.

The first sentence of the 21 CFR 820 Quality System Regulation scope states:

"Current good manufacturing practice (cGMP) requirements are set forth in this quality system regulation. The requirements in this part govern the methods used in, and the facilities and controls used for, the design, manufacture, packaging, labeling, storage, installation, and servicing of all finished devices intended for human use."

In this first sentence, FDA has deemed the topic of methods as not excluded from the purview of FDA. This interpretation is evidenced by the warning letters and Form 483's issued to Medical Device companies described in later sections of this chapter.

Per FDA CDRH, the additional validation related definitions are:

Installation qualification: establishing documented evidence that process equipment and ancillary systems are capable of consistently operating within established limits and tolerances.

Process performance qualification: establishing documented evidence that the process is effective and reproducible.

Product performance qualification: establishing documented evidence through appropriate testing that the finished product produced by a specified process(es) meets all release requirements for functionality and safety.

Where process results cannot be fully verified during routine production by inspection and test, the process must be validated according to established procedures [820.75(a)]. When any of the conditions listed below exist, process validation is the only practical means for assuring that processes will consistently produce devices that meet their predetermined specifications:
Method validation as a requirement is not called out specifically; the FDA has issued warning letters and 483s in relation to the lack of "Method Validation".

W.H.O. Guidance

The World Health Organisation issued draft guidance for Test Method Validation of in vitro diagnostic medical devices in December 2016. Technical Guidance Series (TGS) for WHO: Guidance on Test Method Validation of In Vitro diagnostic medical devices TGS-4
The guidance defines the terms verification and validation as follows:

"Verification is the documentary proof that particular specifications have been met. When designing and developing an IVD, relevant attributes such as cost, and those for performance such as precision, sensitivity and stability are identified and given numerical specifications in design input documentation. It is subsequently the role of the R&D department to design an IVD that will meet those specifications.

The R&D department consequently identifies valid test methods to demonstrate that the specifications have been met (verification) in the new design. Once design has been established, further numerical specifications are produced by the R&D department to ensure that the specifications of each attribute will be met consistently in routine production to ensure quality manufacturing. These new specifications are assigned to control critical production points and may include those for acceptance of raw materials, in-process materials, cleanliness of equipment, qualification of instrumentation and for the finalised IVD to verify its manufacture.

Again, it is also the role of the R&D department to identify appropriate test methods to monitor these specifications. An example of verification is related to incoming goods inspections; each time a raw material is purchased its properties will be verified against the specification using a validated test method."

Validation is the documentary proof that the particular requirements for a specific intended use can be consistently fulfilled. Validation is defined as "verification against needs for a specific use" (i.e. the specification for that use). Within this guide, consistency is essential: it is an expectation that every lot of an IVD will behave as all other lots and will continue to meet design inputs. To ensure this, it is necessary to have validated test methods for measuring and/or monitoring specifications that will consistently produce results fit for purpose. The test methods must be validated to ensure that the results of measuring and/or monitoring are meaningful. For example, the need for accurate measurement of a raw material weighed in micrograms will not be achieved by using a weighing device with tolerance measured in grams. A test method using such an instrument would not be valid for the intended use. Thus, for the example provided, a test method should be specified that has the necessary accuracy and precision for measuring such weights, and an instrument and procedure identified that will consistently achieve this requirement during its use. The test method is then validated to produce results fit for purpose.

Validation of a test method is distinct from its characterisation. Characterisation is documentation of some or all of the features of the method; validation is ensuring that the relevant characteristics are appropriate for the specific intended use. Validation of a method to be used widely, and for standard methods, often begins with complete characterisation. However, for each specific intended use it is likely that only a subset of the characteristics will be relevant and must be evaluated.

ISO 13485, Medical Devices Standard

ISO 13485 is the quality management standard of choice for manufactures of medical devices. Revised in 2016, ISO 13485:2016 "specifies requirements for a quality management system where an organisation needs to demonstrate its ability to provide medical devices and related services that consistently meet customer and applicable regulatory requirements."1 The scope of the standard can apply to any organisation or company involved throughout the life-cycle of a product, including design and/or development, production, storage and distribution, installation, or servicing of a medical device and design and development or provision of technical or professional services.

The recent revision is designed to address recent developments in quality management and other updated regulations that relate to the industry. Improvements in the new version of the standard include broadening its applicability to include all organisations involved in the life cycle of the product, from the concept stage to end of life along with greater alignment with regulatory requirements and post-market surveillance including complaint handling.

ISO 13485:2016 is also used by suppliers or external vendors that provide QMS related management system- services. Requirements of ISO 13485:2016 are applicable to organisations regardless of their size and regardless of their type except where explicitly stated. Wherever requirements are specified as applying to medical devices, the requirements apply equally to associated services as supplied by the organisation. If any requirement in Clauses 6, 7 or 8 of ISO 13485:2016 is not applicable due to the activities undertaken by the organisation or the nature of the medical device for which the quality management system is applied, the organisation does not need to include such a requirement in its quality management system. For any clause that is determined to be not applicable, the organisation records the justification as part of their certification and quality management system.

Basic Definitions as defined in EU Annex IX of Directive 93/42/EEC)

Intended Purpose: Intended purpose means the use for which the device is intended according to the data supplied by the manufacturer on the labelling, in the instructions and/or in promotional materials. (Chapter I section 1 of Annex IX of Directive 93/42/EEC)

Transient: Normally intended for continuous use for less than 60 minutes.

Short Term: Normally intended for continuous use for not more than 30 days.

Long Term: Normally intended for continuous use for more than 30 days.

Invasive Devices: A device which, in whole or in part, penetrates inside the body, either through a body orifice or through the surface of the body.

Body Orifice: Any natural opening in the body, as well as the external surface of the eyeball, or any permanent artificial opening, such as a stoma.

Surgically Invasive Device: An invasive device which penetrates inside the body through the surface of the body, with the aid of or in the context of a surgical operation.

Implantable Device: Any device which is intended:

- to be totally introduced into the human body or,
- to replace an epithelial surface or the surface of the eye, by surgical intervention which is intended to remain in place after the procedure. Any device intended to be partially introduced into the human body through surgical intervention and intended to remain in place after the procedure for at least 30 days is also considered an implantable device.

Medical Device: means any instrument, apparatus, appliance, material or other article, whether used alone or in combination, together with any accessories or software for its proper functioning, intended by the manufacturer to be used for human beings in the:

- diagnosis, prevention, monitoring, treatment or alleviation of disease or injury.

- investigation, replacement or modification of the anatomy or of a physiological process.

- control of conception which does not achieve its principal intended action by pharmacological, chemical, immunological or metabolic means.

A medical device may be assisted in its function by the following means:

Active Medical Device: any medical device relying for its functioning on a source of electrical energy or any source of power other than that directly generated by the human body or gravity.

Active Implantable Medical Device: any active medical device which is intended to be totally or partially introduced, surgically or medically, into the human body or by medical intervention into a natural orifice, and which is intended to remain after the procedure.

Custom-Made Device: means any active implantable medical device specifically made in accordance with a medical specialist's written prescription which gives, under his responsibility, specific design characteristics and is intended to be used only for an individual named patient.

Device Intended for Clinical Investigation: any active implantable medical device intended for use by a specialist doctor when conducting investigations in an adequate human clinical environment.

Intended Purpose: means the use for which the medical device is intended and for which it is suited according to the data supplied by the manufacturer in the instructions.

Putting into Service: means making available to the medical profession for implantation.

Where an active implantable medical device is intended to administer a substance defined as a medicinal product within the meaning of Council Directive 65/65/EEC of 26 January 1965 on the approximation of provisions laid down by law, regulation or administrative action relating to proprietary medicinal products (6), as last amended by Directive 87/21/EEC (7), that substance shall be subject to the system of marketing authorisation provided for in that directive.

Where an active implantable medical device incorporates, as an integral part, a substance which, if used separately, may be considered to be a medicinal product within the meaning of Article 1 of Directive 65/65/EEC, that device must be evaluated and authorised in accordance with the provisions of this directive.
ISO 13485 & Regulations

In Europe, EN ISO 13485:2013 helps companies meet the requirements of: Directive 93/42/EEC on medical devices. This harmonised standard gives companies the "presumption of conformity" to complying with directives.

EN ISO 13485 was published in February 2013 and harmonised in August 2013 to cover the three directives:

90/385/ECC– The Active Implantable Medical Devices Directive (AIMDI)
93/42/ECC – The Medical Devices Directive (MDD)
98/79/EEC – In Vitro Diagnostic MDD (IVDMDD)

Overview of Standard

ISO 13485 has 8 Clauses or Sections which make up the structure of the standard.

Section 0 Normative References, Definitions and Terms
Section 1 Requirements of the Quality Management System (QMS)
Section 2 Normative References
Section 3 Terms and Definitions
Section 4 Requirements of the Quality Management System (QMS)
Section 5 Management Responsibility
Section 6 Resource Management
Section 7 Product Realisation
Section 8 Measurement, Analysis and Improvement

With regard to Test Method Validation, the relevant areas of ISO 13485 include:

(1)   Clause 7: Product Realisation- Section 7.3 Design and Development

(2)   Clause 8: Measurement Analysis

Clause 7: Product Realisation- Section 7.3 Design and Development:

Design and Development Verification and Validation ensure that the product is designed, developed and subsequently manufactured meeting all the customer requirements, regulatory requirements and business requirements. These requirements are classed as inputs to the design and development, and verification and validation ensure the inputs have been adequately taken into account.

The design and development testing sometimes replicate the commercial applications of the medical device, hence providing a realistic challenge in order to have confidence in the medical device.

Design Control

Design control is a necessary practice that ensures good engineering principles are maintained throughout the design phase of a product. It also refers to the continual design and development of the product through its very lifecycle. The design and development files and history must be controlled and maintained, with any changes properly assessed, tested and documented.

Clause 8: Measurement Analysis:

Clause 8 includes:

8.1 General requirements
8.2 Monitoring and measurement
8.3 Control of nonconforming products
8.4 Analysis of data
8.5 Improvement

8.1 General Requirements

Measurement, analysis and improvement are the key themes of clause 8. As with all medical devices, inspection and testing both during manufacturing and post manufacturing is necessary to ensure products and services function as intended and without defects. With any type of measurement or inspection analysis, the method used to complete the testing is critical. The method must be fit for purpose, and the equipment must be suitable. This "method validation" typically is done during the design and development phase.

8.2 Monitoring and Measurement

Monitoring and measurement are dependent on the information or feedback provided from various sources. The most important feedback is the post-production feedback that is gathered from customers or the end user. Again, this occurs over the whole lifetime of the product or service in question. There are a number of methods that can be used to obtain feedback. Some examples include:

-Customer surveys
-Customer complaints
-Review of regulatory databases such as MAUDE.
-Repair and servicing information

8.3 Control of Nonconforming Product

Non-conforming product presents a risk to patients or users of medical devices. When a situation arises where non-conforming product is manufactured or detected through inspection processes, the product must be controlled and segregated to prevent unintended use or distribution.
Some examples resulting in non-conformance are:

- When a manufacturing process drifts outside its validation window or operating parameters.
- A certificate of analysis for a raw material is not provided by the supplier or the results are out of specification.
- In-process testing was not completed at the defined intervals.
- Training of personnel completing tests is not current or is inadequate.

8.4 Analysis of Data

In any engineering activity, data and the quality of the data is a key factor in making the right decisions. Provided the data collected is relevant and accurate, analysis of data can provide important insights into process performance, quality control and product functionality. Data should be collated in a consistent way and controlled by a procedure. When it comes to medical device manufacturing, the sources and types of data are multiple. Data can be generated from in-process testing and data can be generated from end of line testing aka finished product testing.

8.5 Improvement

ISO 13485 fosters a culture of continual improvement. As we have seen, each activity can be described as a process. For example, a manufacturing process, a procurement process, a complaints process. The set of processes that make up the quality management system need to be continually reviewed to ensure they are suitable and effective for the task at hand. Typical tools used to keep improvement in mind include:

- Review of the quality policy and quality objectives
- Frequency and category of corrective and preventative actions (CAPA's)
- Customer complaints
- Management review input

Definitions and Key Concepts

Attribute: is defined as the result of a property or characteristic. It is generally used with the terms pass or fail.

Accuracy: can also be defined as trueness. An expression of the closeness of agreement between the value that is accepted, either as a conventional true value or an accepted reference value and the value obtained. A system with low bias implies good accuracy and vice versa.

ANOVA (Analysis of Variance): a statistical method used to evaluate the significance of differences in means due to different factor-level combinations.

Bias: The difference between observed "average of measurements" and a reference value; also referred to as accuracy.

CQA (Critical-to-Quality): a property or characteristic with specific nominal value and appropriate limit and range providing a particular quality attribute.

Critical Process Parameter (CPP): a process parameter that has a direct impact on critical quality attributes.
Dichotomous Variable: an output with only two possible values. Also known as dummy or indicator variable.

Equipment Qualification: establishing documented evidence that the process equipment is suitable for the intended use and is capable of consistently operating within established limits and tolerances under normal operating conditions.

Process Validation: process validation is defined as confirmation via documented evidence that a particular process performs consistently to a high degree of assurance in accordance with predetermined specifications under anticipated conditions.

Measurement Capability Index (MCI): the Measurement Capability Index (MCI) represents the capability of the measurement system. It is used to evaluate the capability of the gauge to classify product against predetermined specifications.

MSA: a study to determine the degree of error involved in measuring the given parameter. The measurement system involves the combination of operations, procedures, gauges, instruments, environmental conditions, people and software.

Precision: the degree of agreement (scatter) between a series of measurements when a method is applied repeatedly to multiple samplings of a homogeneous sample or artificially prepared sample under the prescribed conditions. There are three types of precision; repeatability, intermediate precision and reproducibility.

Range: range is defined as the interval between the upper and lower measurements required. The minimum specified range should be within the equipment range and validated to operate at all points within the range.

Ruggedness (Intermediate Precision): variation on different days or with different analysts and equipment. The extent to which intermediate precision should be established depends on the circumstances under which the method is intended to be used.

Resolution: the smallest unit of measure that can be obtained reliably from a measurement device, also known as gauge discrimination.

Gauge R&R: represents the estimate of the measurement variation. The measurement variation has two components; repeatability or the precision under the same operating conditions (same operator, test method, sample, etc.) and reproducibility or the precision between operators when measuring the same sample with the same gauge.

Variable: is generally the output that is measured.

Validation: confirmation by examination and provision of objective evidence that the particular requirements for a specific intended use can be consistently fulfilled.

New Test Methods

A test method procedure should be created as early on as possible and trialed and examined for completeness and appropriateness.
If new test methods are required, a revision controlled draft should be available for the purposes of the test method validation.

Changes to Existing Methods

If changes to existing test methods are required, a redlined version highlighting the changes should be made available for the test method validation.

Method Transfer

If an existing test method is suitable for the test method validation, a suitability report can be completed to document the suitability and show that all factors have been considered (see attachment 1). However, the test method should have been previously validated. The parameters at which the validation is to be conducted must be within the existing validated range.

Equipment used in a test method must be assessed to ensure the process is within the equipment qualification. All validation testing must be done on qualified equipment. Equipment qualification is therefore a prerequisite of test method validation.

Test Method Ruggedness Study Protocols

Ruggedness refers to the variation, on different days or with different operators or equipment. The extent to which ruggedness (aka intermediate precision) should be established depends on the circumstances under which the method is intended to be used.

An initial ruggedness assessment should be completed to understand the sources of variation. More formal ruggedness studies may be required which should be captured in a formal study protocol.

The output of any ruggedness studies should detail any changes or modifications to the test method procedure. Generally, a scoring system is used to describe ruggedness which forms a ruggedness assessment. As a result of ruggedness studies and consequent updates to the procedure, the ruggedness assessment needs to be reassessed. This reassessment should be reflected in the final scores of a Ruggedness Assessment Matrix.

Accuracy

Accuracy is a measure of exactness of the test method output or another way of putting it is the closeness of agreement between a set of test results. For example, take a component that weighs exactly 4 kg according to an NIST traceable scale. If the weight of component is taken 10 times on the balance under study using the test method under study then calculate the mean weight of the 10 readings. The offset between the mean weight and the 4kg "accepted reference value" is a measure of bias.

A large bias = poor accuracy. A small bias = good accuracy.
It is important to note that accuracy does not address the variation between individual measurements.

Simply put, if the average is very close to 4kg, then the test method could have been declared to be very accurate.

It is advised that you consult any relevant standards (e.g. ISO, ASTM) to the product or feature being measured as standards often will call out an accuracy requirement. Generally, results should be accurate to ±1% of the measured value. Therefore, the equipment must be fit for the intended purpose or the measurements in mind.

Note: instrument or equipment accuracy can normally be found on calibration certs provided by the manufacturer or vendor.

Precision

The precision of a method is the degree of agreement among individual test results when the same test method or procedure is applied repeatedly to multiple samplings that represent a population.

Precision can be a measure of either the degree of reproducibility or of repeatability of the method.
Repeatability refers to the use of a method using the same operator/test person with the same equipment. Repeatability should be assessed using either a minimum of 9 determinations covering the specified range for the method (e.g. 3 concentrations /3 replicates each). Reproducibility refers to the use of the analytical method in different laboratories such as in a collaborative study.

Ruggedness

Intermediate precision (also known as ruggedness) expresses differences related to laboratory variation, as on different days, or with different analysts or equipment within the same laboratory. The extent to which intermediate precision should be established depends on the circumstances under which the method is intended to be used. The effects of random events on the precision of the analytical method should be established. The use of experimental design (matrix) may be used to study the effects of typical variation (dominance factors) on the analytical method (e.g. equipment, analyst, days).

Representative/Continuous Sampling

Representative sampling is used to determine overall process performance (e.g. Pp / Ppk), which is more applicable for processes known or suspected as less than stable or not in statistical control. Sampling in this way best determines overall spread, which includes within-time and time-to-time variation.

Below, some examples are given on how to sample representatively:

1.   Sampling over a given time-period: e.g. a tray of product is produced every 15 minutes, the period of interest is a 1 hour interval and the sample size is 40.

2.   Sampling a batch or product lot not assembled in any order: if the product is packed in a tray (without any grouping) then sample from various sections of the tray.

Consecutive Sampling

This type of sampling involves taking one sample immediately after each another for the subgroup or time period in question, and is used to determine process capability (e.g. Cp / Cpk).

Consecutive sampling is used in particular to create control charts where a process is sampled in time order by selecting a subgroup sample consecutively and repeating this sampling over a number of subgroups while in same time order.
This method is typically used when the process is stable as there will be little or no causes of lot-to-lot variation.

Range

The range is defined as the interval between the upper and lower measurements required. The minimum specified range should be within the equipment range and validated to operate at all points within the range.

If an existing test method or piece of equipment is to be used, it is important to determine if the method parameters for the new/modified test method are within the validated range of the equipment qualification. Remember, all validation testing must be done on qualified equipment. Typically, the equipment qualification assessment is documented in the test method validation protocol.

Resolution

We have previously defined resolution as the smallest unit of measure that can be obtained reliably from a measurement device or system.

For example, a Vernier callipers may have different models with different resolutions. Some will have only two digits to the right of the decimal point (X.XX mm) and other models could read three digits to the right of the decimal point (X.XXX mm).

The instrument resolution should be better than the resolution of the product specification. If the product specification is X.XXX, then at least a "four-digit" measurement device should be used.

Probability Of False Alarms P (Fa)

This signifies the likelihood of rejecting a conforming unit. This is typically an acceptance criterion for attribute tests. Refer to MSA template for further illustration.

Probability Of Misses P (M)

This indicates the likelihood of accepting a non-conforming unit. This also is typically an acceptance criterion for attribute tests. Refer to MSA template for further illustration.

Validation Protocols

Typically, an approved template is used to create a validation protocol. The protocol sets out the approach to the validation i.e. the approach to qualify the test method. Refer to the appendix for an example of a validation protocol template.

Attachments to the protocol should include ruggedness assessments completed and references to supporting studies/reports. The drafted or "redlined" test method should be attached to the protocol also. The type of MSA protocol (attribute or variable) should also be determined in the validation protocol.

What Can Impact the Accuracy of a Test Method?

Accuracy is influenced by both the instrument (scale) and the test method. If you drop the object on the scale and take a reading before the scale has stabilised, the accuracy is likely to be poorer than when using a test method that demands allowing the scale to stabilise.
Examples include: Tensile strength at break - strength does not exist as a material property independent of the test method used to measure it.
For properties like time, distance, and mass, there are NIST traceable standards that can be measured. These standards have a generally accepted reference value that can be compared to the observed readings to assess accuracy (bias). No such reference sample exists for tensile strength at break, deflation time or implant radial strength. For tests without a reference value, the accuracy of the underlying sensor (e.g. load cell) used to determine the output should be addressed if possible.

MSA Studies

A measurement system analysis (MSA) is an experimental design used to identify the elements that affect measurement variation. There are two types of data in which MSA studies can be completed i.e. variable data and attribute data. These terms are defined below.
Variable data: data that can assume a range of numerical responses on a continuous scale. Most measurements yield variable data.

Attribute data: data that represents the absence or presence of a characteristic.

Non-destructive tests: test where the measured characteristic is not altered due to testing. Since the sample is not altered, multiple readings can be taken on the sample with the expectation of getting the same measured result.

Destructive tests: test where the measured characteristic is changed due to testing. Since the sample is changed, there is no expectation of getting the same measured result over multiple readings.

So, in summary that makes up four types of MSA studies:

- Variable / Non-Destructive
- Variable / Destructive
- Attribute / Non-Destructive
- Attribute / Destructive Table

The following sections describe the requirements, measurement capability indexes and the typical acceptance criteria per MSA type.

General MSA Requirements

Test Environment Conditions - the test environment (i.e. temperature, humidity) should represent the conditions going forward. The effect of multiple environmental conditions can be evaluated if the study is properly designed and planned.

Sample Range - samples should cover the expected range of measurements.

Standard (for attribute MSA) - define the true answer (pass or fail). The standard is based on the inspection ratings of an expert opinion or a measurement system with known better inspection capability than the one under evaluation.

Measurement Instructions/ Training - follow the inspection instructions as defined in the controlled documents or redlines included with the protocol. Do not minimise variability by adding special instructions not defined in the controlled documents or redlines included with the protocol. Reference the controlled documents in the protocol. Special instructions are allowed when using pseudo samples provided that the variability is not minimised due to the instructions. Testers should have a high degree of skill and experience. Do not use new personnel or inexperienced people to conduct measurement studies.

Equipment Qualification and Calibration – The equipment must be calibrated prior to conducting the study. Evidence of the calibrated state should be documented in the report (e.g. calibration certificates etc.). It is important not to re-calibrate the equipment during the study as results can be different due to the calibration effect. The effect of calibration can only be evaluated if the study is properly designed.

Randomisation –

1.   Assign the samples to the first operator in random order. Operator measures the parts.

2.   Assign the samples to the second operator in random order. Operator measures the parts.

3.   Assign the samples to the third operator in random order. Operator measures the parts. Repeat the process described in steps 1 to 3 with the operators for a second and third trial.

Data collection - when documenting the results of a trial, the operator should not have access to the results from the previous trials. A different data collection sheet must be provided for each operator involved in each trial. In lieu of a different data sheet, a data recorder may be used to blind the data recording operator to the test data of previous runs.

Variable MSA Studies

Non Destructive/Variable Msa Studies

The key requirements for non-destructive and variable MSA studies include:

No. of Operators – at a minimum, 3 operators should be used during the study. More operators are also recommended if human/operator interaction is a source of measurement error.

Sample Size – a minimum of 10 units is recommended.

Trials - a minimum of 3 trials should be completed.

Destructive/Variable Msa Studies

If a test is destructive in nature, repeated measurements cannot be taken as the sample is damaged or destroyed as part of the test. One solution is to adopt standardisation of units where homogeneous samples are created by standardising the material or manufacturing process.

- No. of Operators – 3
- Sample Size – 10 units
- Trials – 3 trials

This equates to 90 measurements in total. If standardisation is not feasible, the use of non-destructive pseudo-samples can be used. However, equivalence should be demonstrated between the pseudo sample and "true" units.

Attribute MSA Studies

Non destructive

The recommended and minimum sample size requirements for attribute/non-destructive MSA studies are shown below:

Recommended Minimum Sample Size Requirement

- Operators - 3
- Sample size - 25
- Trials – 3

Destructive

When the test is destructive, repeated measurements cannot be taken as the sample is destroyed or altered. Some approaches are outlined below in order to quantify the measurement variability for destructive tests.

Standardisation Approach: homogeneous and representative samples are created by standardising the method of sample preparation, or material.

Sub-samples: cut each sample into three sub-samples to represent the three trials.

Pseudo-samples: create non-destructive pseudo-samples, documenting a rationale justifying the equivalence of the pseudo samples to the true samples.

Measurement Capability Index

The Measurement Capability Index (MCI) is calculated to assess the capability of the measurement system. The MCI is calculated as a % tolerance.

Measurement Capability Index acceptance criteria:

This index is used to evaluate the capability of the gauge to classify product against the specifications.

The index represents the % of the tolerance (upper specification limit (USL) and the lower specification limit (LSL) that is consumed by the measurement system variation. Figure 9 shows a graphical representation for this index.

Suitability for Use Reports

If an existing test method can be used with no or minor changes, a Test Method SFU Report can be used to document the test method validation.

Suitability for use report is appropriate only if the new product test method parameters are within the existing validated range.

If the test method parameters for the new product are outside of the validated range, the test method must be re-validated. Examples of cases which can utilise such suitability for use reports include:

Test method transfer to a new manufacturing site.
- o New product where the product specifications fall within the validated output range.

o Minor changes in component material which do not impact the validated test. Examples of changes that require full validation include:

New products:

o Extension of product sizes that fall outside the validated range.

CPSIA information can be obtained
at www.ICGtesting.com
Printed in the USA
BVHW011248100620
581261BV00005B/253